Reconnecting With Nature

Finding wellness through
restoring your bond with the Earth

Michael J. Cohen, Ed. D.

Ecopress

Corvallis, Oregon

Ecopress

"Books and Art that enhance environmental awareness"

PO Box 2004
Corvallis, OR 97339
Telephone: 1-800-326-9272
Fax: 1-541-791-2809
Email: ecopress@peak.org
Website: www.ecopress.com
SAN:298-1238

Library of Congress Cataloging-in-Publication Data
Cohen, Michael J., 1929-
  Reconnecting with nature : finding wellness through restoring your bond with the Earth / Michael J. Cohen — 2nd ed.
       p. cm.
  Includes bibliographic references.
  ISBN 0-9639705-2-6
  1. Environmental psychology. 2. Nature—Psychological aspects.
  3. Environmentalism—Psychological aspects. I. Title.
  BF353.5.N37C64   1997
  155.9'1—dc21   96-29597
                                                           CIP

Corn plant illustrations by John Cohen

This book was printed on post-consumer recycled paper.

Publication Date: Earth Day (April 22) 1997

Printed in the United States of America
10 9 8 7 6 5 4 3

This book is dedicated to Serena, and to John Cohen for caring and illustrating the work. It is written in fond memory of Harriet Kofalk.

"This fascinating literary work recycles your thinking. Cohen goes beyond simply exploring a relationship between psychology and ecology. He lets the natural world give us new ways to reason and consciously participate in our relationship with nature within and around us. His optional activities provide discovery, education and emotional support as you do them. Even youngsters learn, enjoy and teach reconnecting with nature through the Internet."

---Chuck Lynd, CompuServe Education Forum Administrator

"This treatise is critical thinking as if nature mattered. The author presents a profound sensory ecology tool that implements the visions of Theodore Roszak, Daniel Quinn and James Redfield....Wendall Berry, too."

---Dr. Daniel Levine, Superintendent of Schools,
Lopez Island, Washington

"Reconnecting With Nature gently blends wholeness and critical thinking. It offers the powerful dimensions of intuition and sense of place to those who want to support responsible action toward the natural world. The multisensory chapters are plain fun, involving both adults and children...skillfully connecting our minds with our experiences and opening our awareness to the lessons of nature."

---Shann Weston, Oregon Project WILD

"I've watched Dr. Cohen's reconnecting process deeply influence and fulfill people's lives. It's a wonderful contribution to healing personal and global relationships."

---Minor Lile, Director
Camp Indralaya
Eastsound, Washington

If the higher purpose of literature is to provoke thought...then Michael J. Cohen has written a masterpiece! "Reconnecting With Nature" is as provocative a book as this reviewer has seen. One of its purposes is to show how to let nature place its wisdom and spirit into our thinking and overcome our separation from its intelligence.

Dr. Cohen presents the case that we have separated from nature's nurture and that is the root cause of our maladies and discomforts. Worse...our natural abilities have been significantly reduced by our society. We live our lives in cement and steel structures that have greatly reduced our appreciation and respect for nature and all that nature offers and teaches.

Thus, "Reconnecting With Nature" is about awareness...and enlightenment and enablement. Dr. Cohen makes us aware of the situation in a bold, forthright yet compassionate fashion. He then shows us that the circumstance is not only solvable...it is do-able. You see, Dr. Cohen has lived, researched and taught in nature for over thirty-six years, now. Not cement and steel...nature, and so he knows of what he writes. He then gives us simple, practical solutions to enable us to find our way back to the loves, truths and integrity that some of our Native American forbearers lived, daily.

Reconnecting With Nature is a waker-upper! Michael J. Cohen has sounded the alarm, defined the problem and given us the tools to put out the fire. This eye-opener is a brilliant self-help book for all seeking renewal in our relationships with our environment, and our selves!

Richard Fuller, Senior Editor
Metaphysical Reviews

Foreword

Recent medical studies affirm what many of us already know: Walking is an excellent way to maintain your health. As Walking Editor for *Prevention* Magazine, I've professionally and personally spent years looking for ways to inspire people to take walks. During this quest, I discovered the reconnecting with nature work of Dr. Michael J. Cohen. I explored its applied ecopsychology by using his book **Reconnecting With Nature** and by enrolling in a fascinating, distant learning course, "Educating and Counseling With Nature," that used the book as its text. People on the course daily shared with each other their experiences with the book's chapters and activities. Mike's nature reconnecting work put a new spirit into my own walks, and into the lives of the six participants in my learning group. It was extremely worthwhile.

The seven of us that did this book together loved its outcomes chapter by chapter. We, and other students, kept a record of what was important to us about each chapter and activity in **Reconnecting With Nature**. If these chapters and activities have half the value to you that they had to us, you will surely savor this extraordinary book, yet they convey only part of what was imprinted on our hearts. Now, when I take the time to reconnect consciously with my surroundings, I'm aware of a whole new way of relating; a way that is both relaxing and stimulating. Walking helps us slow down enough to reconnect with ourselves.

Reconnecting With Nature helps us enlarge that sense of self to Self.

---Maggie Spilner
Walking Editor/*Prevention* Magazine

Acknowledgments

Portions of this book are adopted from the author's published or forthcoming articles in Counseling Psychology Quarterly; The Journal of the Oregon Counseling Association; The Humanistic Psychologist, American Psychological Association; The Science Teacher, National Science Teachers Association; Legacy, Journal of The National Association for Interpretation; The Journal of Environmental Education; The International Journal of Humanities and Peace; Adventure Education, Journal of the National Outdoor Education Association; ERIC CRESS, ERIC SMEAC, ERIC CASS of The U.S. Dept. of Education; Proceedings of the 1987-91 North American Association for Environmental Education Conference and its Monograph of Environmental Problem Solving; Proceedings of the 1991 and 1992 International Conference of the Association For Experiential Education; School Science Review, Journal of the Association For Science Education; Environmental Awareness, Journal of the International Society of Naturalists; The Trumpeter, Journal of Ecosophy; Forum, Journal of Educators for Social Responsibility; The Communicator, Journal of the N.Y. State Outdoor Education Association; Taproots, Journal of the Coalition for Education Outdoors; The Interpsych Newsletter; Cooperative Learning Magazine, International Association for the Study of Cooperative Learning; and Between The Species, The Schweitzer Center of San Francisco.

A special thanks to the following friends for their enthusiasm and involvement in creating earlier editions of this manuscript: Larry Kurtland Davies, Mark Brody, Linda Copes, Steve Smith, Jan Goldfield, Joan Morrison, Gert Braakman, and Lorena Tamayo.

The author is indebted to the dedicated efforts and contributions of participants in Project NatureConnect's support groups. I deeply appreciate following people for sharing their experiences and best thinking about these chapters and activities: Clifford Knapp, Dorothy Austin, JaneAnne Jeffrie, Mike Gintowt, Johanna Jones, Ernie Denny, Heidi Worminghaus, Judy Mac, William Ganschow, Sea Franklin, Mira Fink, Carol Biggs, Barry Fraser, Vicki Seastrom, Rick Raymond, Maggie Spilner Brockman, Linda Copes, Steve Smith, Joan Morrison, Gert Braakman, Larry Kurtland Davies, Mark Brody, Harriet Kofalk, Kathy Doris, David Laing, Joyce Sobel, Eric Thiel, Shann Weston, Jim Sweet, Alice Hibberd, John Roney, Liz Francis, Wanbli Sapa, John Powell, Arja Kaisa, Carol Swan, Christy Andrews, Claudia Robinson, William Byle, Tommy Loggins, Neil Blumenfeld, Teresa Wilson, Rodney Marracci, Nikki Tate-Stratton, David Graham, Ruth Schneider, Elisabeth Ryland, Bob Hobson, Peter Durea, Dorothy Argent, Kathy Brideau, Emmon Bodfish, Don Rittner, Lisa Marks Mahon, Arthur Foster, Forest McCarthy, Doris Jeffries, Ron Slabough, Daniel Levine, Jon Hoyt, Michael Mahaffey, Nils Christianson, Richard Schneider, Terry Anderson, Mark Walsh, Tom Slomke, Peggy Savanik, Jan Veltman, Ken Tohan, Ellen Haas, Jean Anstine.

Finally, I want to acknowledge Serena Lockwood, Jan Goldfield, and Gaia Davies for lending editing and administrative expertise.

Table of Contents

Introduction   11

Part One: Why Think Like Nature?
Chapter 1. Experience the Best Teacher   17
Chapter 2. The Thinking Revolution   19
Chapter 3. Nature's Maverick Genius   23
Chapter 4. Thinking As If Nature Mattered   29

Part Two: Reconnecting With Natural Senses
Chapter 5. How Nature Works: The Wisdom of Natural Senses   37
Chapter 6. The Powers of Natural Senses   53
Chapter 7.   Replenishing Earth and its People: The RWN factor   63
Chapter 8.   Reconnecting With Nature   67
Chapter 9.   People and Nature as Community   73

Part Three: Elements of Applied Ecopsychology
Chapter 10. The Greening of Psychotherapy   89
Chapter 11. The G/O to G/G Formula   99
Chapter 12. Disconnection and the Tropicmakers   111
Chapter 13. The Psychology of Nature Negatives   123
Chapter 14. The Natural History of Personality   137

Part Four: Reconnecting With Nature in Action
Chapter 15. Outcomes   153
Chapter 16. An RWN Activist Speaks His Peace   167
Chapter 17. Self, Meet Yourself   181
Chapter 18. A Chapter of Your Life   189

Appendices:
Appendix A. Transitioning to Nature-Centered Thinking   193
Appendix B. A Case History of RWN   201
Appendix C. An Ecology of Spirit   215
Appendix D. Well Mind, Well Earth by Michael J. Cohen   227
Appendix E. References and Bibliography   229

Introduction

A Moment of Truth

As we begin to learn about reconnecting with nature, we begin to discover why the world works beautifully, yet often does not feel that way in our lives. Nature beautifully sustains itself in balance by using 53 natural senses that we inherit. Our problem is that we learn to restrict ourselves to only five of the natural senses we are born with. The disastrous personal, social and environmental results speak for themselves. Research shows that we can choose to rejuvenate all of our inborn natural sensitivities and make things better.

I recently watched these natural senses perform their magic with a group of informed, caring people. They were insensitive to the value of the performance and chose to ignore it. Their dismissal is cause for great concern.

The performance occurred at a hurried, stressful training session for dedicated community leaders. Their differences kept them arguing amongst themselves. In the midst of this hubbub, a young, wild bird flew into the meeting room through the open door and could not find its way out. Without a word, the behind-schedule meeting screeched to a halt. In that moment, the bird triggered deep sensory attractions and feelings for its life. Hope filled each person. For ten minutes that frightened, desperate little bird catalyzed those seventy people to harmoniously, supportively organize and unify to help it find its way out unharmed. Yet when they accomplished this feat, these people cheered the accomplishment and their role, not the bird's. Its impact went unnoticed. They returned to the hubbub of the meeting, as if nothing special had happened.

I wanted to point out to this group the powerful, energizing, unifying and mutually supportive effect the bird had upon them individually and collectively. Experience told me they would scoff, as they had previously. They would say what had happened was not important or useful since it was uncommon to have a wild bird interrupt their lives.

Unconsciously, these people's sensitivities allowed a touch of nature's plight (a bird at risk) to unite them, to free them from the stress they were feeling and catalyze community amongst them. Although it said not a word, the bird was an educator and counselor. It reached and ignited people's inborn nature. It touched senses of nurturing, love, empathy, community, friendship, power, humility, place, reasoning and a score of others. A bird brought joy, unity and integrity to their lives. The benefits were evident. I have found that it is the lack of such contact that creates and sustains our runaway disorders.

The bird impacted the conference because, as part of nature, it was a part of everybody at the conference. Humanity is to nature as our leg is to our body. We are one, an integrity that is sentiently unified. For example, as we breathe Earth, Earth breathes us. Its life is as dependent on the air we exhale as we are on the air it produces. Our desire to breathe is a specific natural sense, a love for air. We did not invent that love. It is of, by, and from nature. We inherit it and many other attraction sensitivities from nature.

The bird reconnected us with nature. It sparked some of our natural sensations and feelings into consciousness and things came out right. Anybody can learn to create similar experiences that afford similar outcomes. We don't do this because long ago we learned that to expressively enjoy and validate nature's ways was similar to having an illicit affair.

Our lives don't make sense and our problems flourish because industrial society does not teach us to seek, honor, and cultivate nature's contributions to our lives. We learn instead to conquer, to separate from and deny the time-tested love, intelligence, and balance found in the natural world.

Reconnecting With Nature Activities
A Hands-On Learning Option

The natural world, including our inner nature, contains attractions that intelligently hold it together and sustain it in balance. The activities in this book enable the reader to consciously connect with these attractions in nature and you.

Participating in the activities lets nature's intelligence show your mind that it is reasonable to enjoy and benefit from nature-connected thinking. It is attractive.

The reader has the option to read this book straight through or use the chapters as supportive reading for hands-on experiences with nature. You may accomplish this by doing the activity, located at the end of each chapter, before you read the chapter.

Although the nature reconnecting activities are simple to read, reading them is like reading an instruction manual for driving an automobile. To have the car take you where you want to go, you must actually drive it. To have the activities reconnect you with nature, you must participate in them. Do them in conjunction with an attractive natural area: a park, backyard, or even a potted plant. The activities enable your verbal-reasoning mind to reconnect with your sensory mind while it is connected with nature's ways. This connection enables you to think with nature. If you participate in the nature reconnecting activities, the chapters become exciting adjuncts to your first-hand experiences. They also help build relationships if you share them.

For best results, be sure to do the activities at least a day apart. This lets your sensory inner nature grow, nourished by dreams, while you sleep. You awaken with new insights and feelings. The chapters will repeat some points that otherwise might be forgotten due to the sleep time interjected between them.

Important: For reasons that will unfold through the book, the activities are specifically designed to work with things that you like about nature, that attract you at the time you are doing the activity.

If something you are attracted to becomes unattractive for any reason, (for example: it arouses fears, bad memories, negative stories, or discomforts such as weather changes) immediately seek a new aspect of nature that is attractive at the moment.

If an activity does not work for you, try it again later when it feels attractive to repeat it. Sometimes when you are already enjoying a strong connection with nature, an activity may feel like an interruption. Don't do it until it feels attractive. Sometimes an activity becomes attractive when you decide to learn it to help another person reconnect with nature. You will find that you get as much out of teaching others these activities as you do from learning them for the first time. They become your personal gift to those who seek nature's rewards.

We are accustomed to letting people help us learn through verbal communication. If you share your thoughts and feelings from doing an activity with another person, an important part of your mentality will validate your activity experiences. This increases your experience's credibility and benefits. Verbally sharing your experiences, thoughts, and feelings from the activities is as valuable as the nature connections the activities provide.

Activity numbers and chapter numbers are identical. For example, activity 6 is found at the end of chapter 6.

You may read and learn a great deal from the reactions of others to the activities. They are found on our internet appendix page:

http://www.pacificrim.net/~nature/appendix.html

I invite you to join our internet mailing list to contact others who will share in your activities and vice versa. It is described on our contents page: http://www.ecopsych.com. This book is the text for our introductory courses located at this Internet site.

Part One:
Why Think Like Nature?

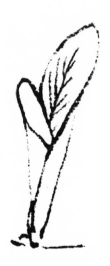

Chapter One

Experience the Best Teacher–Nature

Each of our 53 natural senses is a distinct feeling experience

We are born of nature. We emanate from a natural biological expression of love between our parents. However, nobody ever asked our permission for us to be born. We neither selected our parents nor consented to become part of our culture, creed, language, nationality, or social system. However, we live in, and are shaped by, the envelope of each of them. There is no question that they mold how we think, how we see and relate to the world. Are you satisfied with their effects? Do the effects of how we learn to think make sense? Many people believe we can do better.

On average, most people are not satisfied with the impact of our way of life. They see that it is not as healthy as it could be, it does not sustainably support life. For those who seek ways to increase wellness and reduce our adverse effects, I offer the process of reconnecting with nature.

From early on, the authorities in industrial society shape us to live physically and mentally separated from nature and its balance. Our nature-estranged way of life is not the only way to think and live. It is the way that has happened to us. Thankfully, we are given the freedom to choose. If we are attracted to a more nature-centered way of life, it is reasonable to choose to become closer to the intelligence, beauty and peace found in nature. When given the opportunity, that's what most of us do. That is why most of us flee to natural areas on vacation and when we retire. Our vacation is an attempt to vacate our problem-stricken daily way of life. Our problems are absent in intact natural areas. Unlike us, nature thrives and grows through life-supportive relationships. It is simple for us to learn how to involve ourselves in nature's way, for it is already part of us. We simply have to unbury it in ourselves and each other.

Activity 1. A Chapter Of Your Life

This book builds on your attraction experiences in nature. It enables you to obtain their benefits at will. I encourage you to start the process by writing your own chapter here. To the best of your ability, write a paragraph or two about the most attractive experience you can remember having in nature. It may have taken place while you were alone or with others. It may have been in a park, your backyard, or a wilderness area. It could have been with a pet, an animal, plant, or your surroundings.

If you think you have never had a good experience with nature, write a paragraph about why you think you would like to have one.

Once you have completed writing the paragraph about your attractive nature experience, answer the following questions about them:

1. What sensations made the experience attractive, enjoyable or rewarding?

2. Were you taught to have the worthwhile sensations in your nature experience in a class? From a book? Wasn't it your inborn natural sensory attractions to the natural area that provided the enjoyment and rewards?

We are biologically constructed to sense natural attractions. Your most attractive experience in nature consisted of many distinct, different sensations such as temperature, color, and touch. Hunting and gathering societies find that following their natural sensory attractions in people and the environment is a key to survival in balance. We each inherit this ability. Have you ever considered giving thanks to Nature for it?

Find this ability in yourself by going to an attractive natural area such as a park, backyard, beach, or potted plant. Note that some aspect of this area calls to a sensory part of you that appreciates it. This is a biological natural attraction connection between you and this natural area. You naturally sense it, it is a love that is alive and well in you. The sensory attraction invites and welcomes you to be there, it feelingly encourages you to enjoy this moment. On a sensation-feeling level it gives you permission to be here. Can you thank it and your sensory self?

Now, use your sense of language to further validate that attraction experience by putting it into words. Write a statement that says to the effect "I know that my inherent sensitivities to natural attractions are alive and well because when I visited this attractive natural area, I could enjoyably sense and feel _____" Include what you sensed: colors, forms, shapes, textures, pressures, temperatures, fun, motion, emotions, etc. Note that you can have these same sensations and feelings about people, too. Although they exist without verbal language, they are a form of connectedness shared throughout nature. Do you trust them?

Chapter Two

The Thinking Revolution

Nature connected thinking uses 53 sources of sensory information

If you are missing out on the natural joy and wisdom of life, it is because you have been taught to ignore it. If you have enjoyed even one good experience in nature, you know what potentials you are missing by not having those good feelings most of the time. A visit to a natural area shows that nature approaches perfection when it comes to intelligently living in harmony. Nature is an excellent model that does not display our runaway problems. Think about the experience you described in chapter one. Do you recognize that you did not have to learn how to enjoy its rewards? Your potential for experiencing them is built into your soul and biology. They automatically take place when you connect with the natural world. Learn to sustain its rewards, and Earth, by learning how to let similar experiences in nature teach you to think like nature works. You are born as nature with this knowledge intact. You can use it and remember it by reconnecting with it.

Chances are you have not heard of this scenario: an unheralded coastal island where people enjoy their beaches, gardens, woodlands and community friendships. Unlike elsewhere, most people are satisfied with their lives. They feel relatively safe and content.

People who know of the island do not identify it for the same reason that its residents refuse to give it an official name. This prevents it from being discovered and overrun by those who are attracted to its virtues but do not know how to help sustain them. That could happen, it has happened elsewhere.

The island's population has already achieved far lower than average rates of stress, crime, drug-use, disease, pollution, divorce and abusive relationships. Problems always arise, but the inhabitants support each other and protect the land while solving them. The natural environment there exists in balance with the island's ability to sustain personal and natural integrity. Property values continue to rise. This island lies within 100 miles of three major population centers.

Servicing its visitors makes a major contribution to the island's economy. The island's population sustains itself partially by careful contact with the many millions of individuals who want to enjoy and learn the unique nature-connected thinking process by which the island population achieves its happy balance. The waiting list of people who want to visit the island steadily increases. When people visit, they come away owning the ability to enlist nature's wisdom in their lives. No matter what their occupation or age, most island inhabitants have the ability to teach this rewarding process as it applies to them and their interests. I know farmers, teachers, ranchers, parents, politicians, business people, students, health and social service workers who enjoy and share the process with others.

The island built and owns its own airport, bridge, parking lots and ferry service. It regulates the number of people that may use them. The revenue from their use pays for most government services. Inhabitants enjoy a strong sense of community and lower than average tax and health insurance rates.

The particular island I have in mind is, in part, a fantasy. However, I created and teach the ecologically sound educational and psychological thinking process by which many pockets of people and places achieve the island's integrity. Although industrial society's thinking downplays them or tries to change them, islands of humanity like this exist throughout the world. You can learn their nature-connected thinking process. You can learn how and why the process works and how you can easily inject it into your life and community. If you care to learn and apply it, you will gain the personal and professional expertise to create and enjoy "island life" and introduce its qualities to others.

Reconnecting with nature consists of bringing into your consciousness a sensory way of thinking and relating with which you are born. Moment by moment, throughout nature, it produces consensual relationships at every level, from microorganisms to natural people to weather systems. It is the process that nature uses to sustain its diversity, peace, and sanity. The life-sustaining integrity, beauty and intelligence of nature demonstrates that it works. Our challenge is to follow our natural attractions to achieve nature's integrity. We can choose to learn how to mindfully reconnect with a global process that brings the good feeling of cooperation and wisdom of nature into our thinking.

Every species, including nature-centered human cultures, think while in resonant contact with nature's intelligence. Their mentality works like nature works, for it is part of nature. For this reason, they live in a continuum with nature's ways. Industrial society teaches us to think differently. Its premise is that for our society to exist, we must think in ways that subdivide and conquer nature within and around us in order to build our excessive indoor world. Authorities in society wrangle and program us to think in disconnected ways while we are powerless as children. We have little choice. We learn to reason and live in a story and process that promotes an undeclared, hidden war against nature. It victimizes us as we learn to conquer nature and crush its intelligence within us.

When we destroy any integrity beyond its capacity to regenerate, the integrity disappears. Today, we live with the disastrous effects of sacrificing the integrity of nature. Without nature's guidance, our minds are distorted. As exemplified by the bird at the conference, when we come in contact with nature's integrity, we seldom recognize, accept, or honor it. The state of the world shows that, disconnected from nature, we have not the intelligence we need to resolve our runaway personal, social, and environmental problems. Our thinking is mentally deficient when it is nature deficient. However, enough of nature remains to recycle our thinking and restore personal and global integrity. Master the secret and let nature-centered thinking catalyze that restoration.

Activity 2: Partnering With Nature: A Discovery Experience

Go to something in nature that you like, that you find attractive. A park, a backyard, an aquarium, or a potted plant will do. When you get to it, notice how you feel. Can you thank it for your good feelings?

Now, treat this area fairly, with respect, as an equal or friend. Don't bully it, instead gain its consent for you to visit and enjoy it. Ask this natural area for its permission for you to be there. Doing this increases your sensitivity to the area. Ask it if it will help you learn from it. You cannot learn if you are going to injure or destroy it, or it you. Wait for about half a minute. Look for adverse signals of danger such as thorns, bees, cliff faces, etc. If the area still feels attractive, or becomes more attractive, you have gained its consent. If this portion of the natural area you visit no longer feels attractive, simply select another natural part that attracts you and repeat this process. Do this until you find an area where a safe attraction feeling remains for 10 seconds, then thank it.

Once you have gained an area's consent, compare how you feel about being there now with how you felt about it when you first arrived. Has any change occurred?

If you find that gaining a natural area's consent to visit it is rewarding, remember that you can do this, or any other of the book's activities, whenever you want to become more connected to nature.

Here are some reactions of past participants to this activity. Add your reaction(s) to the list. Share them with others:

"It was hot. Soon after I asked for permission to be with the grove of young trees, a gentle, refreshing breeze came through them. It cooled me, and the trees waved their leaves at me. It felt good, like the grove smiled its consent."

"I was attracted to the sound of a raven on the rocks ahead. I stopped and sought its consent for me to enjoy its presence. It began to come closer and closer, increasing my fun and excitement. That was unforgettable."

Write down important things you learned from this activity. Write down what good feelings may have been brought on by doing this activity. To discover this activity's effect on your sense of self, complete a sentence that begins with: "My experience in Nature shows me that I am a person who gets good feelings from _____". Use this sentence form whenever you connect with a natural attraction. It reinforces a positive, natural self-image.

Chapter Three

Nature's Maverick Genius

*Our multisensory nature contains a consciousness that
we share with the natural world.*

The road to civilization does not necessarily lead to the runaway clutter and destructive ways that mark industrial life. To find a better road, our thinking must be attracted to return us, in reality and imagination, to our origins in nature and society. From them, knowing our past errors, we can make enjoyable, responsible choices to natural attractions. They lead to additional enjoyable, responsible moments and their attractions. This process carves a path that our children and others can follow. The path molds them to continue building that path.

To return our thinking to our origins means going back to basics. The "basic" we most need is trust in ourselves, our natural attractions, and our environment. The most trustable truth in our life is the safest place to start building additional attraction relationships we can depend on. However, when I ask people to tell me the greatest truth in their life that they can trust, they usually come up with the wrong answer. Our blind rush to "get ahead" has usually blinded us to the correct answer. The right answer is neither God, love, nor honesty. Although this sounds brash, seldom do people disagree when they learn the "right" answer. My "right" answer is that for each of us, the most trustable truth in our lives is our immediate experience. For you, it is that you are reading these words right now, or that you can feel the seat you may be sitting on or the shoes on your feet. Our immediate experiences are the closest we can get to a trustable reality. For example, when you feel thirsty, that is a trustable reality. It is an authentic attraction to water, not a fantasy. If we can't trust the immediate experiences that we sense, what can we trust? In the immediate moment, we can always check what we sense in many ways to see if it actually exists.

If we do not activate and support sensations from direct contact with nature in the moment, we do not trustably return to our origins in nature. Instead, what we know are stories about nature from the past. These stories are often not fully accurate, since nature changes and stories are often only partially reflect this. Stories are not nearly as trustable as what we directly sense in the immediate moment.

Our personal reality in any given moment consists of our natural sensitivities registering on our screen of consciousness. That is the time we can think with these senses and relate to and through them. That is when we can consciously connect them with nature. For example, if your inner nature signaled that you were thirsty in this moment, would your thinking trust that sensation's message? Would you trust your sense of thirst, the signal that your system was attracted to drink water? Would you decide to drink? Would you act from that decision and take a drink? Would that be a reasonable relationship to have with your sensory inner nature and the water in the environment?

The immediate moment is the only time that nature actually exists or that we can consciously change our relationships. For example, it is only in the moment that we feel the attraction called thirst that we can choose how and what to drink.

When we react only to the images, memories or projections that play in our mentality, we fill the moment with feelings and reactions to stories, old pictures, and the sensations attached to them. We relate to past experiences, not to the realities and potentials of the immediate moment. Life only exists in the present. Everything else is images, labels, and stories.

Reconnecting with nature activities help participants recognize the natural potential of the immediate sensory moment. You might try doing this "in the moment" activity and see what it teaches you:

Pinch yourself and recognize that the feeling you experience in this moment is real and true. Can you trust that you feel it, that it is a way of your nature consciously knowing and expressing this moment? That sensation of touch and pain is a natural contact with reality that has biologically and psychologically evolved over the eons.

Now stop pinching yourself. Think about what you just did. Note that the experience itself was more real than the memory that you did it. The original experience has become history and our history strongly shapes us to be who we are now. However, in the immediate moment, our history is a story. What we fully are in the immediate moment is what we think, feel, and do. It is not just our memory of past moments, not our fantasies about future moments. It is us in the immediacy of our lives. In our excessive removal from contact with nature, rules and schedules have replaced knowledgeable contributions from our natural senses. That loss results in our loss of natural wisdom, respect and balance.

Note that you can't pinch yourself too hard in the immediate moment. When you do, your natural senses of pain and reason usually bring to consciousness thinking that says: "disregard that you were told to pinch yourself. We do not give our permission for you to continue doing this. Stop hurting yourself with that story. It is attractive to gain sensory satisfaction that is more responsible and rewarding. Do it now." Each moment contains some form of this basic intelligence. It is the genius that guides Earth. Like ignoring the role and impact of the bird at that conference, we have learned to ignore gaining consent from nature.

Instead, we habitually think with stories that exclude nature in the moment. That is our problem, not its solution. Thinking that includes nature's wisdom and consent puts us on a wise path. That path includes the process by which nature governs itself. It helps explain why nature does not produce runaway garbage, war, and abusiveness. Nothing in nature gives consent for them. We produce our troubles by teaching ourselves to avoid that path.

For 35 years I have learned to reconnect with nature, moment by moment, while extensively living outdoors throughout the seasons. Nature experiences, similar to yours in chapter one, have created in me a resonating chamber. Knowledge gained from my studies in biology, education, and psychology, allow me to understand nature in reasonable words and thoughts arising from intimate contact with nature's wisdom and beauty. The process and observations that I share in these chapters are not the tainted product of the same 35 years that I ordinarily might have spent in the warp of stress, mistrust and chaos that ordinarily pervades life at home, work, and school. I have avoided our collective madness. I have let nature teach me, and others, how to continue avoiding it and promote islands of sanity. Anybody that is attracted to doing this can do it. You simply let attractive moments in contact with nature replace the stories within and around you that say you can't do it.

When I went to sleep outside in a forest by the bay last night, I thought about this book and many facets of reconnecting with nature. As I slept, I heard geese sing as their wings whooshed through the air. I heard otters calling, playing, splashing. I heard the wind sing in the trees. As brilliant stars burned above, a doe and fawn walked by my bedside. I was aware of this concert on many levels of sleep.

I woke up with the sun this morning. I had one word in mind: salt. Fascinating, isn't it? Why salt? Because of a fascinating story: I have heard about an infant who said the word salt very early in life, long before he could say anything else. He said salt many times, nothing else, just salt. Sadly, the baby died. The autopsy revealed the cause of his death to be a salt deficiency.

It makes no difference whether the story of the salt-deficient child is true. To me, the salt message I awoke with is clear. Reconnecting with nature last night by sleeping outdoors reminded me to tell you about that salt deficient child. As I describe reconnecting with nature to you, you may stop and wonder, just like you would wonder if you heard that infant say salt. You see, nature is a marvelous intelligence that sustains the integrity of our living planet, but that our current nature-separated thinking has little use for. Nature's intelligence is as foreign to our nature-disconnected thinking as an infant saying "salt." It is, no doubt, unusual for you to hear me say "Nature is a marvelous intelligence, a maverick genius, that speaks to us every moment of our lives through at least 53 natural senses."

Sometimes dealing with nature's sensory impact on us makes people think that they are disturbed or the world is crazy. For example, people are attracted to being happy, but can't find happiness. They relish responsible relationships, but can't build them. I teach educational sensory nature activities that enable people to become conscious of nature in the immediate moment. Participants thoughtfully reconnect with nature's incredible wisdom, beauty, and integrity. Responsible, enjoyable thinking and relationships, on every level, result from this attractive process. It is sane and that simple.

This book lets nature say "salt" to you and others in every field of endeavor, in every aspect of your life. Reconnecting with nature enables you to know how and why you may locate, respect, and respond to nature's intelligence. This is a wisdom we each biologically inherit, one that enriches every minute of our lives as we become conscious of it. Because our society is estranged from nature, our leaders do not teach you that skill. Many refute it. However, you may easily learn it, just as I did, directly from nature. It can happen in your backyard, a park, or the back country. Without a majority of us having this skill, we ignore a vital personal and global knowledge that nature within and around us offers moment by moment.

The skills of reconnecting with nature are worth learning. It can avoid disorders, just like the ones the salt-deficient child suffered. He suffered due to people's lack of knowledge about his salt deficiency. Our alarming negative social and environmental indicators show that we suffer because we are nature deficient. We can learn to hear attractive and wise sensory messages from nature within and around us. We can learn how to consider them and respond to their creative guidance. But, if you listen hard, you will not hear nature saying the word salt. It says the word love. It says we suffer a vast deficiency of natural love and it says how and where that love may be found. Nature can teach us that love for it is key to our happiness. However, be aware that nature teaches its love through sensory attraction experiences in nature, not by using words. Nature is non-verbal. Each natural attraction experience is a form of love. The natural world involves a type of love that neither uses nor understands verbal language and stories. Can part of you trust that? That part is your inner nature.

Activity 3: Being There

The idea that nature and our inner nature contain intelligent love frightens many of us. In chapter five, we will learn that we can know and learn through 53 natural senses. Each is a natural intelligence. The nature-separated way that we learn to think overrides them.

To know how to swim, sooner or later you must want to get into the pool. To truly enjoy nature's intelligence, you must want to experience your natural senses. Cognitive awareness of them alone is not enough. Why not get in the pool now? Feel them. Before going any further in this book, go to a nearby attractive natural area, the more natural the better. If necessary, a potted plant, an aquarium, or a square foot of lawn or earth will do. As you did in activity 2, ask for the natural area's permission for you to visit and become involved with it. Gain its consent to help you with this activity.

The natural world involves a type of love that neither uses nor understands verbal language. Can part of you trust that? That part is your inner nature. To help discover and enjoy non-verbal nature including your inner nature, take ten minutes or more to enjoy this natural area's attractions in silence. Each attraction is a mini-love. During this ten minutes ask the natural area: "Who are you without your names and labels?" Wait for some kind of response to come into consciousness. Then ask: "Who am I without my name?" Again wait for some response to occur. Repeat this procedure for ten minutes or more as long as it is attractive. The following are some responses that others have had, can you learn from them?

"This was fun, nature became the attractions I felt for it, and I became them, too."

"Without labels, everything became active and alive."

"Things became their essence. Rocks, tree-beings, sensations, and spirit."

Write down what you experienced during this visit and its value. Do you know this natural place and/or yourself differently now than before you did this activity? Recognize that the place never said a word. You may have converted the experience into words, but the natural area never said them. Write down a few things that were important to you about this activity and chapter. Write down what good feelings may have been brought on by doing this activity. How would you feel if your ability to experience them was taken from you? Do you trust these feelings as being real? What effect does this activity have on your sense of self-worth?

Chapter Four

Thinking as if Nature Mattered

Each of our 53 natural senses is a distinct way of knowing, loving and feeling.

What is your 39th natural sense? Do you use it when you think? If not, your thinking is probably not as "sensible" as it could be. That may be the source of some of your problems and those of the world as well.

The disturbed state of Earth and its people suggests that our thinking suffers from a deficiency. From early in life we learn the habit of paying attention to things industrial society considers important. In the process we lose sight of "unimportant" realities. For example, note that being able to read this sentence is important civilized behavior. As you read it, in this moment you are conscious of its words and phrases, not its individual letters. Yet it was individual letters that held your attention before you learned to read. Now they have little meaning. Now that I bring this phenomenon to your attention, you are probably conscious of the individual letters on this page in this moment. However, this will cease shortly as your normal reading habits resume. When we habitually learn something has little meaning, we lose sight of that thing until we break the habit.

The disappearance of individual letters from our consciousness as we learn to read resembles what happens to the value of nature and our natural senses as we learn to live excessively separated from the natural environment.

Even though you are born with dozens of different natural senses, you have learned to ignore them to the point that you probably don't even believe they exist. You instead believe Aristotle who, in the cradle of our civilization 2500 years ago, theorized the existence of 5 senses: touch, taste, smell, sight and hearing. However, the truth of life is not only what Aristotle or our civilization says, but also your own natural attractions, thoughts, and experiences. For example, when you feel hungry you are attracted to food. Do you trust that you actually sense hunger? Most people do feel this sensory attraction, yet the natural sense of hunger is not one of our acknowledged five senses. Neither is the natural sense of excretion, nor gravity, nor motion, nor are the natural senses of community, place, and consciousness. These natural sensitivity attractions pervade nature and us. They are each a form of natural intelligence. It is extremely intelligent to want to eat when your body needs food!

You may have been taught to think it is unreasonable for you to believe that you have an 18th sense. But that in itself shows that you have a sense of reason and the sense of reason is one of our 53 natural senses. You are involved with the senses of language and consciousness at this moment. Each of these natural senses is a distinct, different, inherent way of knowing; touch is different than smell, conscience different than gravity, language different than pain. For the past 50 years, researchers have clearly established the existence of at least 53 natural sensitivities in people and nature.

We each inherit nature's ability to sense and make sense in at least 53 different ways. However, unlike nature-centered cultures, our civilization does not help us sustain this natural wisdom in our consciousness so we are often not aware of it. Never the less, nature, including nature-centered people, uses all of these senses to organize, preserve, and regenerate itself. Through these sensitivities nature wisely creates its optimum of life, diversity and beauty without producing our garbage, war or insanity.

Because society teaches us to overlook nature's attractive natural intelligence in ourselves and nature, we don't learn to validate or use it. However, empirical demonstrations show that when we reconnect to nature through our natural senses, we psychologically plug into nature's intelligent ways. They do not contain or promote stories as such because they use sensory attractions, not verbal language, to communicate. Our bodies respond to these attractions and we become conscious of nature's wisdom. This helps explain why problems often melt when we visit natural areas. It is more than just getting away from our problems. It is going to a place that people did not invent, a place whose intelligence does not generate, support or fuel our problems and has shown to diminish them.

Unlike our way of thinking and its questionable personal and global effects, nature's intelligence does not continually undermine itself with "Yes, but" stories. These stories have us spend most of our lives reasoning or arguing with other stories. Remember, nature's intelligence has no stories. It is illiterate. It thinks by trusting and combining the innate intelligences that lie in its natural attraction loves. That creative, trusting way of thinking has thoughtfully sustained, balanced and evolved the natural world's perfection for eons. We are born knowing that thought process. If you find it reasonable and attractive to explore it, don't let your own, or others, "Yes, but" stories stop you from participating in these activities and chapters. These pages help you learn from nature to thoughtfully, habitually connect with its intelligence in your inner nature.

The following reconnecting with nature activity lets nature introduce you to parts of itself in you. If this invitation feels honest, reasonable, and attractive, trust this moment. Permit its attractiveness to guide you. Continue to learn how to incorporate nature's intelligence in your thinking.

Activity 4: The Sensory Nature Walk

This activity works best and has more interesting results when done with a partner. However, the next to last paragraph describes how to do it by yourself.

Often we are habitually conscious of the world through the following three senses:

1. Sight
2. Language
3. Reason

Our highly trained and educated 3-sense perceptions often overpower our other awareness abilities. This leaves our consciousness and thinking devoid of our many other non-language, sensory ways of knowing and being. For this reason, it makes sense to produce some nature-connected moments in which we may thoughtfully discover and experience, first hand, many other natural ways of knowing that we inherit from nature.

Go to a safe, attractive, natural area. As you did in previous activities, ask for this natural area's permission for you to visit and become involved with it. Gain its consent to help you with this activity. The activity lets you sense the natural world using your less developed natural senses. It asks you to share a safe natural area with a partner as follows.

Without talking (minus language), one of the two of you close your eyes (minus sight). The other person becomes a nature guide who holds your hand and in other appropriate ways supports you. If it is safe, you may take your shoes off.

The nature guide's responsibility is to, in as many ways as possible, safely and gently introduce you to the natural world in this area. The guide requests that you imagine you have just walked off a spaceship into the unknown, or just have been born onto Planet Earth. This disconnects your sense of reason, for in your imagination you are like a newborn baby where everything is new.

For five minutes be led by the guide to sense, touch, feel, taste, smell, roll in, crawl through, hug, and occasionally see glimpses of the many different natural parts of this area that the guide selects to fulfill his or her mission to safely introduce you to nature. With respect to using the sense of sight, the guide can move you close to any natural entity and place you in any position or angle. The guide can focus your closed eyes on natural attractions he or she sees. The guide can signal you to open your eyes (only for a second) by squeezing your shoulder, and then releasing it to signal you to close your eyes again. This balances the use of sight with the use of other senses. Practice doing this quick eye-opening procedure before you start the activity.

After doing the activity for five minutes switch roles with your guide. You guide him or her.

Some things guides might want to have their partners do (without talking):

- If it is safe, have partners remove their shoes.
- Smell, hear, and momentarily see the soil, flowers, leaves, tree trunks, and moss.
- Hear the rustle of leaves, the sound of the wind.
- Feel the warmth of the sun.
- Look up a tree trunk, at natural things close and far away.
- Roll down a gentle embankment.
-Hug a tree, lie in leaves or grass.
-Face different directions, towards and away from the sun, the wind, or different sounds.
- Walk across interesting terrain.
- Have an ant walk on their skin.
- Gently place their face on leaves, rocks, or just feel the wind.
- Hear a brook, bird, or insect.
- Lean over to be aware of gravity.
- Gently have the inside of their wrist feel a thorn, water, sand, grass, or a spiderless web.
- Feel your pulse, your breath, temperature changes, the inside of your mouth, your hair, their ear, their nose.

If you can't find a partner, or for added information and fun, do this same activity solo. Find a safe natural area and with your eyes closed, explore it for five minutes. Walk, creep, and crawl around to guide yourself as described above, opening your eyes only for a second every few steps. Be sure to do this activity with a partner at some point. It offers something extra that way.

What are your thoughts, feelings, reactions, and sensations as a guide? As one who was guided? What natural senses (sensations) did this activity bring into your consciousness ? How did they feel? Did you want to put names on things or identify them? Write down your experiences. Share them with your partner and others.

Here are some things other people have sensed doing this activity. Did you experience them to any degree?

"I trusted my partner more; found new ways to balance; sensed community; had fun; know this place differently; was hungry; sensed more intensely; things looked more brilliant; felt supported; liked the adventure; had a hard time not labeling things; sensed fear; lost track of time; liked communicating non-verbally; became aware of design and textures; intuited where things were; became more relaxed and alive; hardly recognized myself; sensed responsibility for my partner."

In the next chapter, you will learn about a list of natural senses people have felt while doing this activity.

Write down the three most important things you learned from this activity. Write down what, if any, good feelings were brought on by doing this activity. How would you feel about not being allowed to have them? Did this activity enhance your sense of self-worth?

If you are interested, you may read the reactions to this activity by several other people who have done it and posted their results to their international study group via e-mail at the following web site: http://www.pacificrim.net/~nature/appendix. Be careful. Do not measure yourself against these responses. I only post them so that readers may get some idea of the potential that lies in these activities. Each of the other activities contain the same potential.

Part Two:
Reconnecting With Natural Senses

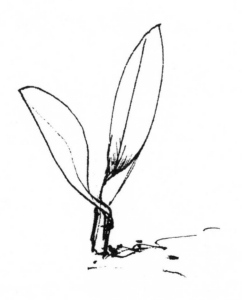

Chapter Five

How Nature Works:
The Intelligence of Natural Senses

To disavow any natural sense is to play the role of an ignorant god.

Although life and death are two phases of the same process, we sense them as opposites. We are alive, we prefer life because our life and all life is attracted to live. We know we are alive because we have a sense of consciousness. It acts like a movie screen in our mind. Our screen of consciousness has things appearing on it. For example, these words you are reading now are registering on your screen of consciousness. You are conscious of them, so you know you are alive. When there is nothing playing on the screen, or the screen itself disappears, we say we are unconscious or dead. We could truly say "I am conscious of thoughts and feelings, therefore I know." The screen of consciousness itself is one of our 53 natural senses that we inherit. We sense consciousness. There are 52 additional natural senses that, when energized, register on the consciousness screen. Each sense is a vital, distinct way to know life and to be alive. Each exists in some form throughout nature.

Nature Centered Consciousness
Human beings learn to survive as conscious beings. We train ourselves to know the world by what appears on our personal screen. Often we don't differentiate between the words and stories that appear on the screen and sensations and feelings that register there. For example, if we are in a movie theater that presents a frightening murder story, we register the story in our sense of consciousness and we feel frightened. It is as if a real murderer stalks us, even though we know it is just a story on a theater screen. Unless we reason that we should focus on the moment and bring into consciousness that a murder movie is just a story, the mental images that register in consciousness have the same power to bring up sensations and feelings as does a firsthand experience. I demonstrate this phenomenon to my workshop participants by telling them I am going to get them to salivate by having them taste a lemon. I tell them I will peel the yellow skin off the lemon, slice the lemon into thin juicy pieces, and

pass them around on a plate. Each participant is to first smell their lemon slice, then taste it, and then squeeze it into their mouth and drink the sour juice. Before I ever get the lemon out, participants who have previously tasted a lemon are already salivating just from my words (and so am I). Perhaps you are, too, if you have had past experiences with a lemon. This exemplifies how our story effects us in the same way that a direct experience does. The difference is that we usually can't do anything to change the past experience or movie/story itself. However, we can choose to involve ourselves in a different story or experience at any given moment.

Sensory Reality

Nature centered psychology recognizes that it is reasonable to be conscious of all our natural senses and sensations, not just our stories. Our sense of reason can discern that it is reasonable to let our inherent natural intelligence be nurtured by nature, provide pleasure, and help reverse the troubles of our personal and collective lives. We must learn that it is reasonable to do this and how to do it. For example, I ask people to pinch their arm so it hurts just a little and then to hug themselves or stroke their cheek in a way that feels nice. In questioning them about these sensations, they say that they that they recognize these feelings are real and they trust them. Their ability to feel sensations is not just a fantasy. They also say they know and trust that other people feel, that sensations and feelings are facts in the lives of others. When somebody says they feel something, it is believable that they do. Participants say they sense that the ability to feel is present in people no matter what their culture or location on the planet; that people 10,000 years ago had the ability to feel and that people 100 years from now will have it, too. Many even say they are sure that animals and plants have the ability to sense or feel on some level. In other words, it is common knowledge that our feelings exist in the immediate moment, the ability to feel has been around for a long time and that we trust it across boundaries of people, time, distance, cultures, and perhaps species, too.

Sensory Unconsciousness

Reconnecting with nature activities help people validate what they sense and feel in the immediate moment. Too often our unnurtured sensations and feelings escape our awareness. Our attention is wrangled away from what we immediately know and feel to stories we have been programmed to pay attention to. For example, as you read this paragraph, it is the words and phrases that catch your attention, you don't actually register the white space in between the letters, or the page itself. Perhaps now you do because I call them to your attention, but your reading habit will again shortly focus your attention on the words here. This domineering phenomenon makes the following question puzzle even scientists, educators, and psychologists when I present it to them:

"Like every other living thing, people are part of the water cycle. Water from the environment comes into us, through us, and out of us. What do you know that makes water do this? Also, what regulates the flow of water through us so that we don't bloat or explode from taking in too much water, or dehydrate from too much water leaving us?"

Most people feel they are not qualified to respond to the question. Those that do usually say things such as: "Water flow in people is determined by biologic osmotic pressures and salinity factors." Sometimes they say: "Cell membrane qualities and homeostasis regulate water flow," or "God made it so."

Rarely does anyone mention that the natural sensation of thirst is a contributing factor to having water flow through us, yet we each have known since childhood that thirst plays that role. Thirst is nature's way of telling us to drink. Most of us are wrangled to depend upon knowing when to drink through our stories, our education. We don't drink when we are thirsty, we drink by meal time or break time schedules, by the availability of water or flavors added to it. Like this page's white space, we lose consciousness of what we naturally sense. In this case it is thirst, a natural sensation we have known since birth. In addition, most participants do not state that their sensation of thirst is also a water regulating factor that prevents them from bloating or dehydrating. We learn to forget that thirst "magically," "intelligently" appears when we need water. As we drink water the feeling of thirst "magically" subsides because it is naturally intelligent. It has the sense to recognize that our need for water has been satisfied, so it turns off the call for water. We are often more conscious of the language based idea that the formula for water is H2O. Similarly, we disregard that our sensation of excretion is intelligent. It has the sense to tell us to return water to the environment. It is not that we don't know these things, it is that we learn not to pay attention to our old brain feelings. This is similar to our discovery of how much sense our sense of touch contains when we do activity 4.

What society wrangles our new brain to know about water as a chemical and scheduled resource becomes more important than what we innately know through our natural senses. It is as if our story about a lemon has replaced the importance of having a real one. But, the story of the lemon won't prevent scurvy just as a picture of water won't prevent thirst. We can't drink or prevent scurvy with our stories about water or a lemon, we need the real thing.

Our society's story mostly teaches conquest and improvement of nature, not sensitivity and respect for it. We learn to overlook the nature connected wisdom of our many lifelong sensory ways of knowing, like the wisdom of thirst. We don't learn to honor the roles and properties of thirst in supporting our lives. In this way our nature-separated lives mislead us. We lose many possibilities for our lives to enjoy the natural intelligent relationships that pervade the biological world and sustain it in balance.

The sense of thirst exemplifies the properties and fate of each of our many other inherent natural senses. However, when we remove the invalidating names we give them and directly experience them as sensations, we discover that each sense is a distinct natural sensation unlike any other. Even though they contain nature's cohesive ability to blend, thirst is different than community, which differs from color, which differs from hearing. On our screen of consciousness, each sense has the potential to register its self-governing, balancing contribution to personal and global life. Each sense will do so if our thinking allows it to appear in consciousness. We have educated ourselves to mostly be conscious through new brain stories. We must teach our sense of reason to respect that each natural sense presents a feeling whose story is as important and real as the things it connects. The sensation of thirst is as important and real as water.

Nature connected consciousness

Nature reconnecting activities reverse our sensory omission. We learn from experience by doing them. They bring into our nature-deprived consciousness the importance of our inherent sensory ways of knowing. For example, the blind walk, activity 4, teaches participants how to temporarily turn off their story signals. Once these signals are quieted, participants become conscious of many other natural sensations and connections that constantly call to them. They not only feel these sensations, they learn to validate their existence by describing them. They become aware in language of how good these senses feel in nature, and how this feeling replaces stress that they formally felt. They discover that, just like the sense of thirst makes sense and feels good when fulfilled, each of their dozens of other natural senses also make sense and provide good feelings when fulfilled. They discover that ordinarily their nature separation stories hold their attention and thereby deprive them of their common sense, their full spectrum of natural sensory intelligence and good feeling. They discover from their personal life experiences how society teaches them to lose their respect and dependency on thirst and water for survival, and how it may be replaced by commercial products, for example, Coca-Cola® (The Real Thing?!®). They discover that they have become addicted to nature replacements for survival and good feelings (Things go better with Coke®).

As I write this chapter, an e-mail has come from somebody in the USA doing the blind walk activity. I offer their letter here as an example of what happens in nature when we grow into using natural senses we usually ignore:

Hi Interact Group Friends:
I did this activity right after dinner and initially I was feeling a little reluctant to get out of my indoor 'womb.' But the moment I stepped out into my backyard everything changed. This turned out to be a very powerful experience for me. I was led with my habitual senses turned off and I was surprised that the mere act of not speaking and closing my eyes changed my total perspective. Everything felt intensely sensual and I felt that my senses became keener. Sounds felt magnified. I heard the chirping of a mockingbird and the squawking of a crow. I sensed forms that I usually overlook. I balanced myself in different ways and felt the texture of the ground. I also wanted to pay more attention to the crackling of my feet walking over the ground cover. I felt motion, temperature changes, gravity, distance, and trust that usually escape me. I felt nurtured in a new way and a greater sense of place and community.

But the thing that struck me the most was the incredible diversity of the textures I experienced through touch. It's like I never realized just how different everything felt, how many ways they could be sensed. When I was lead to the trees, I felt a strong affinity as I touched them. Very strong feelings of life. I felt a strong kinship. A very emotional loving experience for me. Tears came to my eyes.

Later, as the guide for another person, I felt like I wanted to give to my partner the same wonderful experience my partner had given to me. Here is an individual I've been close to for years and suddenly being in the same places sharing natural things that attracted me brought on wonderful new feelings and closeness for both of us.

The overall experience felt like we entered another friendly world, very focused, pure, and clear. I really enjoyed it.

Best wishes,

Ricky

Language addicted consciousness

We innately feel/experience natural senses. These feelings are each unique and we give each of them a name. Too often we lose contact with the love and passions our natural sensitivities carry because we have been taught to know these sensations as mechanical, misleading words such as "emotions," "needs," "drives," and "instincts." However, no matter how we label or define them, nature created these distinct sensations and feelings. It also created our ability to register and store them and the wise nonverbal life experience messages they carry. We increase our ability to register and remember them by assigning them a name that revives them in verbal consciousness. The natural senses and our ability to label them are part of nature and human nature. In addition to ourselves, most species, from minerals to mountain lions, own and react to these same sensitivities in some way. They may not label or feel them as we do, but they react to them. Natural attraction sensitivities cohesively hold the world together and govern it. The world holds them in common while we have been educated to lose consciousness of them. Is it any wonder that we are insensitive to the global community and its callings? It elicits responsible interactions from every other species.

Consciousness, a natural sense, did not come to us from out of nowhere. Like the other natural senses it, too, pervades nature. In people, the sense of consciousness has been given an ally, the sense of language. Language allows consciousness to be more alive and active in people than in most other species. It appears that only humans think through verbal stories. That disconnects us from nature when the stories don't accurately convey our senses or how nature works.

Human consciousness is a registry of natural attractions. Those same attractions create and sustain relationships within atoms, minerals, plants and animals. Our consciousness is naturally aware of the many senses that we feel, for it is one of them. However, our excessively language-trained consciousness often replaces direct sensitivity to other survival senses. This occurs to the point that our stories allow our consciousness to become conscious of itself. We mostly sense in and through language. The sense of reason organizes our words in our consciousness. We call this process thinking. We learn to think in words and images. We treasure and learn to nurture our thinking, our story, about our consciousness screen and what appears on it. However, this does not honor the senses themselves. We are educated to subdue and direct our senses rather than honor them. They are not words, they are sensations. Often they don't register on our word-addicted screen of consciousness. Much of nature thus becomes subconscious.

Sensory Consciousness

Normally, the fulfillment of natural attraction sensitivities, organism to organism, builds and interconnects the natural world as a community. This is the loving wisdom of Earth connecting and communicating (communing). Collectively, the interconnections blend, meld, and ecologically balance to sustain Earth and its diversity of minerals, species, and cultures. For this reason learning how to consciously enjoy, validate, trust, appreciate, and strengthen our natural senses holds great potential for personal and global fulfillment, balance, and unity. In nature centered thinking, it is very important to honor natural sensory communication even though it is mostly nonverbal.

The evolving creation process of the natural world, not humanity, "invented" our natural senses. They originate from nature's cohesiveness as nature's ancient love of life diversifies. For example, an organism living in the sea has little need for sensing the equivalent of thirst. It does not need it because it is surrounded by a matrix of water, an essential of life. But, if an organism evolves as a land animal, a natural survival attraction sense similar to thirst must simultaneously evolve to keep the organism connected to water. The organism's life loves and needs water. Without the sensitivity or intelligence to know it needs water, the organism dies. In order to remain part of nature, an organism diversifying from the matrix must develop the appropriate natural attraction sensitivities to keep it connected to the matrix. These sensitivities make it part of the whole of life. They are essentials of life.

Too often our story based education fails to emphasize the importance of our natural senses. It overlooks that our many natural sensory loves bring onto our screen of consciousness the natural attractions that hold the world together. These attractions keep all of life, including ourselves, alive. Our education wrangles us to lose awareness of our sensory connectedness and support from the global life community. Often we may feel abandoned when we are actually strongly supported by natural sensory connections that we have been educated to disregard. They are invisible to us, buried in our nonverbal subconscious.

Many reconnecting activities let Earth reconnect us and bring these various loves of life to our consciousness as appropriate words. Mark Germine, a psychiatrist and psychological journal editor practices many kinds of therapies including hypnosis. With respect to using sensory nature connecting activities, he says: "I have not seen such a deeply unconscious state brought to the surface before."

We may conclude that as any living organism physically separates from nature's essentials, the life process genetically encodes that being with natural attraction sensitivities to keep it connected to those essentials. In fact, these natural sensory attractions form and sustain our genetic makeup. We experience this network of attraction connections through our many sensory anatomical, neurophysiological, and perceptual attributes.

As does everything else in nature, each natural sense and sensitivity plays a role in surviving. Each signals something special about our relationship with the natural world that exists in ourselves, each other, and the environment. That signal is part of life itself. The communication system of our planet consists of an immediate, growing, ever-branching network of differing connective attractions of, by, and from the creation force in nature. Each natural sense is an intelligence in and of itself. It is wise to use this intelligence to build good relationships.

Nature does not know or use our language. In nature, senses and sensitivities have no name. Although we don't always know how plants, animals, or minerals register natural senses and sensitivities, we do know that we feel them. We label our nameless natural feelings according to how they fit into our new brain stories. Depending on the story in which we are raised, we call them: Attractions, Loves, Sensations, Affinities, Spirit, Resonances, Invitations, Callings, Intuitions, God(s), Great Circle of Life, Communications, Affections, Blessings, Bonds, Higher Power, Natural wisdom, Us, The Nameless, and many others. No matter what we call or label them, our natural senses and feelings are facts. They are attractions, loves as real, true, and provable as are rocks, water, and trees. They are as real as feeling ourselves caress or pinch ourselves. To avoid the stories from desensitized authorities that often control these senses, I sometimes call the natural senses "nameless." Nameless confronts our word-addicted thinking with a reality of life it too often overlooks; nature consists of attraction relationships, not words.

We are normally born with our natural senses intact and healthy. Consciously or subconsciously they thrive until deadened. They constantly seek the pleasure of fulfillment from connecting with their origins in nature. In this way, they avoid the pain of being thwarted, disconnected or unfulfilled. The sensory wisdom of Nature is that in people, the fulfillment of each natural sense produces comfortable, satisfying feelings that also benefit the whole of life. Nonfulfillment produces desires for fulfillment, for sensory satisfaction, for love.

Our natural senses and feelings are our multiple personality, our array of selves, the true nature of our inner child. For us to responsibly enjoy life, each unadulterated natural sense requires our attention, trust, and nurturing. Each natural sense is a beautiful, nonverbal intelligence and love. Each natural sense has value for each makes its special contribution to stability, survival, and sanity. Industrial society has created many contrived   stories that wrangle and amputate these senses from our consciousness and from nature's integrity. In natural areas, participation in the nature reconnecting process reverses this amputation and its adverse effects on personal, social, and environmental relationships.

The Multisensory Person

People may not inherently feel all of nature. We feel only that part which we exercise or which supports our evolutionary survival in the natural world. For example, our sense of sight doesn't ordinarily register infra-red or ultraviolet light, although other creatures do register it. Biologically the creation process may have evolved us to survive without seeing these ranges. Similarly, cats may survive seeing only blue and yellow, and many animals are color blind altogether.

Each of the 53 natural survival sense groups that pervade nature and us are listed below. They help us enjoy and improve our lives. We experience them as an essence of our desire to be alive, as attractive callings that connect nature within us to the natural environment, to other peoples' inner nature, and to global life processes. Through our natural senses we more fully know nature within and about us. The more we awaken, fulfill, and nurture them, the more we sense lasting fulfillment in the satisfaction, balance, and wisdom of nature's peace.

The list below contains general categories of senses. Each sense can be further subdivided. For example, I list color as single sense yet we sense many thousands of colors. Each different color represents a different sensitivity, each may signal a different mood or message, each has different intensities that have different meanings, each may have a different neurophysiology and genetics. For example we consider taste as one sense, but our ability to taste salt, sweet, bitter, and sour are each physiologically, chemically, and anatomically unique. There are 22 different ways to experience touch. Each sense has a different genetic blueprint in us arising from eons of biological experiences and diversifying relationships within the global life community.

Most natural senses are present but unexercised in an infant. Even the sense of reason and place operate in 2-month old babies. Since we didn't invent natural senses, and can't know them solely through language, each natural sense mystifies our thinking. Albert Einstein said: "The most beautiful thing we can experience is the mysterious. It is the source of all true art and science."

Between the years of 1961-1978, researcher Guy Murchie made an exhaustive study. He painstakingly scrutinized scientific studies about the senses as they appeared in many hundreds of books and periodicals during those 17 years. In 1986 he told me that scientific methodology and research had actually identified over eighty different biological senses which pervade the natural world. He said he additionally verified this through authorities at the Harvard Biological Laboratories. All these senses he clumped together as 31 groups for literary convenience in his book The Seven Mysteries of Life published in 1978. His painstaking efforts and bibliography deserve our applause and confidence.

Although Ames, Gesell, Pearce, Rivlin, Gravelle, Samuels, Sheppard, Sheldrake, Spelke, LePoncin, Wynn, and many other researchers continuously validate our multisensory nature, the full significance of it has yet to be recognized by industrial civilization's story. Our intellect thinks that if it has a story about them, then we are OK. Our addiction to our story mediated, nature separated lives and thinking keeps natural senses and their value hidden from our immediate awareness. Our economy fuels itself by keeping our senses discontented, further irritating them through advertising and then selling us products that satisfy them.

Our natural senses are nature in action. They attract us to the whole of the natural world and its ways, including the inner nature of other people. As our society trains our intellect to conquer nature and the natural, we learn to conquer our natural senses. Our nature-disconnected sense of reason exalts the senses that our stories use to take over our other senses and the natural world. We subdue and demean the remaining senses that tell us about how the natural world works and enable us to participate in the process. Ignored and numbed, our natural senses are a vast missing part of a responsible story about Earth, ourselves, and community. Without them registering in consciousness we become "half vast." As Carl Jung and others have noted, our abstract thinking is no more reasonable, logical or consistent than are our feelings. While living in the outdoors, nature has taught me that our abstract thinking is the way we learn to put our natural senses into culturally reasonable stories. Our challenge is to recognize that the excessively nature-separated parts of ourselves and our culture are unreasonable.

We desperately need nature's wise ability to maintain life without producing our problems. That wisdom stops our society's destructive actions against ourselves and the environment. The absence of it from our consciousness is the mother of our collective madness: our runaway wars, pollution, dysfunction, disease, mental illness, apathy, abusiveness and violence. Without nature-centered thinking, our consciousness abandons our sensory inner child. Anybody can choose to help reverse this situation by choosing to learn how to reconnect with nature itself, not abstracted stories or videos about nature.

I offer the following list of natural senses with this important reminder: each sense is a distinct attraction energy, an intelligent love that in nature has no name. Each is aware of itself by its being, not by a name. Each is an experience. Each can awaken many natural parts of us when we use it to connect with the natural world. That touchy-feely, hands-on, connecting experience in nature, not this list, catalyzes personal wisdom, growth, and balance. This list only provides information in language. It brings it on the consciousness screen and feeds and guides our senses of reason and language, our story way of knowing. Reason and language are only 4% of our inherent means to know and love nature, life, and each other.

Nature-centered thinking uses the list of senses in conjunction with visiting natural areas and exposing our indoor conditioning to the many natural senses awakened in nature. It uses the names of the senses to help the new brain validate our natural sensations. Doing this is reasonable, since once we experience a sense, speaking its name places that sensation in our verbal consciousness. There we can think with it. This process non-verbally connects, rejuvenates, and educates us. It allows us to safely extend into the natural world's intelligence in order to more fully sense our lives and all of life. It works because once we experience that process of intelligent love and wisdom, we own it. We never fully return to our former way of knowing.

Natural Senses and Sensitivities
The Radiation Senses

    1. Sense of light and sight, including polarized light.

    2. Sense of seeing without eyes such as heliotropism or the sun sense of plants.

    3. Sense of color.

    4. Sense of moods and identities attached to colors.

    5. Sense of awareness of one's own visibility or invisibility and consequent camouflaging.

    6. Sensitivity to radiation other than visible light including radio waves, X rays, etc.

    7. Sense of temperature and temperature change.

    8. Sense of season including ability to insulate, hibernate and estivate.

    9. Electromagnetic sense and polarity which includes the ability to generate current (as in the nervous system and brain waves) or other energies.

The Feeling Senses

    10. Hearing including resonance, vibrations, sonar, and ultrasonic frequencies.

    11. Awareness of pressure, particularly underground, underwater, and to wind and air.

    12. Sensitivity to gravity.

    13. The sense of excretion for waste elimination and protection from enemies.

    14. Feel, particularly touch on the skin.

    15. Sense of weight and balance.

    16. Space or proximity sense.

    17. Coriolus sense or awareness of effects of the rotation of the Earth.

    18. Sense of motion. Body movement sensations and sense of mobility.

The Chemical Senses

    19. Smell with and beyond the nose.

    20. Taste with and beyond the tongue.

    21. Appetite or hunger for food, water, and air.

    22. Hunting, killing, or food obtaining urges.

    23. Humidity sense including thirst, evaporation control and the acumen to find water.

    24. Hormonal sense, such as pheromones and other chemical stimuli.

The Mental Senses

25. Pain, both external and internal.

26. Mental or spiritual distress.

27. Sense of fear, dread of injury, death, or attack.

28. Procreative urges including sex awareness, courting, love, mating, and raising young.

29. Sense of play, sport, humor, pleasure, and laughter.

30. Sense of physical place, navigation senses including detailed awareness of land and seascapes, of the positions of the sun, moon, and stars.

31. Sense of time.

32. Sense of electromagnetic fields.

33. Sense of weather changes.

34. Sense of emotional place, of community, belonging, support, trust, and thankfulness.

35. Sense of self including friendship, companionship, and power.

36. Domineering and territorial sense.

37. Colonizing sense including receptive awareness of one's fellow creatures, sometimes to the degree of being absorbed into a superorganism.

38. Horticultural sense and the ability to cultivate, as is done by ants that grow fungus, by fungus that farm algae, or birds that leave food to attract their prey.

39. Language and articulation sense, used to express feelings and convey information in every medium from the bees' dance to human literature.

40. Sense of humility, appreciation, ethics.

41. Senses of form and design.

42. Reasoning, including memory and the capacity for logic and science.

43. Sense of mind and consciousness.

44. Intuition or subconscious deduction.

45. Aesthetic sense, including creativity and appreciation of beauty and music.

46. Psychic capacity such as foreknowledge, clairvoyance, clairaudience, psychokinesis, astral projection and possibly certain animal instincts and plant sensitivities.

47. Sense of biological and astral time, awareness of past, present and future events.

48. The capacity to hypnotize other creatures.

49. Relaxation and sleep including dreaming, meditation, brain wave awareness.

50. Sense of pupation including cocoon building and metamorphosis.

51. Sense of excessive stress and capitulation.

52. Sense of survival by joining a more established organism.

53. Spiritual sense, including conscience, capacity for sublime love, ecstasy, a sense of sin, profound sorrow and sacrifice.

This list explains how, sense by sense, nature connects with itself in us, through us, and to people and places around us. It suggests that we can consciously engage in this process. It validates Dr. David Viscott's proposal that feelings are the truth, that we don't live in the real world when we ignore what we are feeling. Our nature-separated lives disengage and de-energize these senses. Notice that the senses of reason, language, and consciousness are three of the 53 senses listed here. We have learned to respect what they bring into our awareness. The language in these chapters and activities suggests that it is reasonable to learn how think and build relationships through all 53 of our senses, not just these three plus the well known five senses. When we attempt to think and relate this way, we introduce a reconnecting with nature (RWN) factor into our daily lives. The RWN factor helps nature, the mother of these senses and feelings, to nurture and strengthen them. This rejuvenates and restores them. The process gives them enough energy to appear on our nature-desensitized screen of consciousness and green our thinking.

Activity 5: Sensory Intelligence, Information and Powers

Do our natural senses and their intelligence deserve our trust? Do they have powers that we use to the fullest advantage?

1. Have in your possession a pencil. Go to a natural area. As you did in the previous activities, ask for this natural area's permission for you to become involved with it. Gain its consent to help you with this activity.

2. Place six or more similarly sized sticks or rocks before you.

3. Shut your eyes and then pick up one stick.

4. With your eyes remaining closed, mark the selected stick with your pencil. Then feel the stick all over until you feel confident that you have familiarized yourself with its shape, texture and other attributes.

5. With your eyes still shut, return the stick to the pile. Mix up the pile of sticks. Now pick them up one at a time and feel them until you believe you have found the stick you selected and marked.

6. Now open your eyes and note if you have selected the stick you marked. Try this a few times.

7. What conclusions can you draw about your sense of touch?

This activity demonstrates the many facets, powers, and connections of a single natural sensory intelligence: *touch.* Each of our 53 senses have similar powers. They make similar contributions to our ability to intelligently know and feel alive.

You can do a variation of this activity in a safe woodland. After getting the area's permission to visit, shut your eyes and have a friend, without speaking, lead you to one tree in the area. As with the sticks, spend as much time as you need getting to know this tree with your eyes closed. Then have your friend lead you away from the tree. Now, open your eyes, go back into the woodland and see if you can find the same tree. Your friend can tell you if you are right, and, of course, so will the tree if you "make sense" with it by touching it.

Write down the three most important things you learned from this chapter and activity.

Write down what, if any, good sensations and feelings were brought on by doing this activity.

Can you describe them? How would you feel about having your ability to feel them taken away?

Does this activity enhance your sense of self-worth?

On our appendix portion of the Project NatureConnect web page, http://www.pacificrim.net/~nature/appendix.html, you may read the reactions to this activity by other people who have participated in it and posted their results to their international study group via the Internet. Caution. Do not measure yourself against these responses, learn from them. The nature of others often brings out the best of our own nature. I include them so that readers may get some idea of the potential that lies in each one of these activities.

Chapter Six

The Powers of Natural Senses

*Our natural sensations, being fluid attractions, meld
with each other to sustain balanced relationships.*

As I note in the previous chapter, most people are surprised to
discover that our natural sensations and feelings are intelligences of, by,
and from nature, This is exemplified by the water attraction and regulator
that they know as thirst, a natural sense. By activating or deactivating like
a control valve, thirst helps regulate and sustain the water flow in our lives
by turning on and off. Similarly, every other natural sense acts as an
intelligent, self-regulating control valve as well. Most people are also
surprised to learn that our sensations and feelings do not belong to us
alone. For example, we and Earth cooperatively experience thirst for our
mutual benefit. It keeps the flow of water going like a bloodstream that
picks up and delivers nutrients wherever it goes. We share the sensation
of thirst with Earth, it is a property of the natural world as well as
ourselves. In this sense, thirst is as much a part of water as is wetness. Our
nature-separated lives blind us to the oneness of our natural senses and
nature. Sensing that oneness is foreign to most of us.

Each natural attraction we feel means one or more of our natural
senses has awakened and their energies have brought them onto our screen
of consciousness. Each is a part of nature within us energizing as it
connects to itself in the natural environment and vice versa. Each natural
sense non-verbally "remembers" eons of life experience for they come
from it. Each is a different expression of life's desire to exist. Each has
valuable powers and makes valuable contributions that, too often, our
stories ignore.

When we feel natural sensations, we actually sense the global life
community nurturing and balancing its flow in and through us, guiding us
as part of it. For example, we have the ability to sense and enjoy the color
red. As humanity evolved, redness contained some important aspects of
survival. For example, red is often the color of ripe fruit. Similarly, with
taste, a fruit's degree of sweetness also discloses its degree of ripeness.

The sweeter, the redder, the more ripe, the more digestible. In addition, fruit usually smells good when it's ripe. The fruit's smell, taste, and energy act as rewards to the multiplicity of senses that enable a natural community to know what, where, when, why, and how to be in the right place at the right time to gather and enjoy the fruit. Most of our natural senses come into play and know how to contribute to fulfilling the sense of hunger. We love fruit. These are not sensory coincidences or irrational, fatalistic ways of knowing and being. They are nature's cohesive attraction wisdom in action. When we validate it, we experience the trustable and enjoyable sensory fulfillment of being in tune with nature and we reduce the stress generated by its unfulfillment. This does not happen when we connect our senses to contaminated or false stories about separating from nature. The stories mislead our inner nature and we end up in our fears and problems.

Life does much of its work on microscopic levels. Eons ago, natural sensory attractions enabled microorganisms to intelligently "invent" or evolve into immensely complex, stabilizing, survival relationships. These include fermentation, photosynthesis, genetic coding, and decomposition. We inherit from nature a multisensory "Velcro"® that continually attracts, attaches, and bonds us to the natural world. Our natural sensory attractions explain why children are infatuated with nature. We don't learn to love pets, fawns, and baby seals. We are born with that love, their presence simply energizes it onto our screen of consciousness. The 53 natural attractions/senses/loves that nonverbally created and sustain infatuations remain alive and well when we exercise, treasure, and celebrate these senses.

By validating the global unity that results from natural attraction forces interconnecting, it becomes reasonable for us to trust that we and nature are one. Validating that atoms and their particles consist almost entirely of attraction forces (natural loves) validates the observation that "Love is the only reality of the world because it is all." The truth of the eons appears to be that the wisdom of nature is love. Love and live could be the same word. Lest this all seem simply an academic matter of semantics, recognize that the meanings we attach to words defines our existence. Thomas Mann offers that speech is the essence of civilization while Elbert Hubbard suggests that we exist because, unbeknownst to us, natural intelligence loved us to be.

Multisensory Intelligence

The power of the natural senses is simply that they non-verbally attract, blend, and share their time tested experiences with each other. That is the source of natural intelligence. It does not discriminate, rather it cooperatively brings all kinds of useful knowledge together in consciousness. When we use it, we call it critical thinking. When intact, natural senses relate to and modify each other. This sensory ability to blend makes it easy and natural for us to change based on how we feel rather than what we have been wrangled to think. For example: Imagine that you go out to eat in an expensive, renowned restaurant. The menu is beautifully designed and everybody's food looks appetizing and tastes great. To your surprise, the waitress brings out your order. Your scrambled eggs are dark brown, the ham is sky blue and the potatoes bright green. Most people feel uncomfortable by this color change and won't eat the food. This color change example demonstrates that each sense touches, influences, and modifies other senses. The natural senses "talk" to each other and thereby make common sense not only in ourselves, but throughout nature. Plants and animals also behave differently when they sense a foreign configuration. This helps determine in the moment who is predator and who is prey. This is part of their sensory history and our own.

In optimum conditions all senses are naturally attracted to support eating, but in this example the unusual food colors, although attractive in themselves, are out of synchronization with past survival experiences that our senses remember. This signals something is wrong. The signal influences the other senses to recognize that something is inconsistent with respect to survival. When this happens, eating becomes uncomfortable, if not impossible. It is no longer attractive. In this example the unusual food colors turn off the natural sensory experiences of place, community, trust, intuition, and others. This influences appetite, touch, taste and smell. It reduces or nullifies them. Until consent is given by all the senses, nature fills in for the shortcomings in a forgiving, non-punishing way. Nature asks us to follow some other natural attraction such as eating a food with an appealing color. Through experiences with nature, our thinking can learn to trust this asset of nature. On a chemical level, this same flow of information and use of logic even exists in biomolecules within cells. Why should this surprise us? Eons ago this flow originated on microorganism and mineral levels and remains intact.

Another example of natural multisensory wisdom is that our thirst is affected by heat (temperature sense), salt content (chemical sense), fatigue, and sight, sound, taste, or even thought (language, reason, consciousness senses) of water. Our thirst is influenced by a congress of senses and it in turn influences other senses. For example, thirst, as it intensifies, activates the sense of pain which in turn calls further attention to seeking fulfillment of thirst or to sensory clues as to where water might be available.

The sensory congress welcomes the contribution of any sensory information, including pain, in order to make sense. In a fluctuating concert, the natural senses form a trustable consensus, a common sense that helps life survive.

As does every other sense, our language and reasoning senses create stories that also color what we know. Ask yourself: would you have eaten the breakfast if the colors were okay but the ham was labeled "grasshopper meat," the eggs were labeled "fecal matter," and the potatoes had a skull and cross bones on them? Labels bias our perceptions, thinking, and behavior. A label or story can either separate us from, or connect us to, nature. For our health and happiness, we must critically evaluate our labels and stories by their effects.

I use an interesting activity to help people recognize the immense power of labels and language on the screen of consciousness. I have a person place two identical teaspoons of equal weight on a table. They then hold their hands out in front of them, close their eyes and imagine that their left hand holds a rope from which hangs an immense, heavy rock. Their job is to try to keep their hands together, and the rock in the air, off the ground. Meanwhile, their right hand holds a rope attached to a large helium balloon which tries to pull their hand skyward almost stretching it. Then they imagine that more rocks and balloons are being added. They remain in this image with their eyes closed for one minute. Then they open their eyes. They note their arms are no longer parallel with each other, they have moved. They pick up one teaspoon in each hand. The spoons no longer feel like they are of equal weight. The spoon in the heavy rock hand feels lighter than the spoon in the helium balloon hand. The discrepancy results solely from the "rock" and "helium balloon" stories I gave them. The stories pollute their ability to perceive the reality of the teaspoons being of equal weight and this all takes place in less than two minutes. Now think about the profound distorted effects produced by living year after year in stories and places that separate us from and demean nature and our natural senses. With respect to nature, we live our daily lives in another world, a separate reality. It is a story world that has been desensitized to nature's callings and balance. Are you satisfied with its effects?

The sense of respiration is an example of our natural sense relationship with the atmospheric matrix. Remember, respiration means to re-spire, to re-spirit ourselves by breathing. It, too, is a consensus of many senses. We may always bring the natural relationships of our senses and the matrix into consciousness by becoming aware of our tensions and relaxations while breathing. The respiration process is guided by our natural attraction to connect with fresh air and by our attraction to nurture nature by feeding it carbon dioxide and water, the foods for Earth that we grow within us during respiration. When we hold our breath, our story to do so makes our senses feel the suffocation discomfort of being separated from Earth's atmosphere. It draws our attention to follow our attraction to air, so we inspire and gain comfort. Then the attraction to feed Earth comes into play so we exhale food for it to eat and we again gain comfort. This process feels good, it is inspiring. Together, we and Earth conspire (breathe together) so that neither of us will expire. The vital nature of this process is brought to consciousness when we recognize that the word for air, spire, also means spirit and that psyche is another name for air/spirit/soul. This is the psyche presently being explored in the field of ecopsychology. Reconnecting with nature activities keep the psyche well by enabling our story to consciously understand and cooperate with nature, to rediscover how that feels. That brings language and reason into the arena. It influences them to validate respiration since they, too, are part of it. For example, our stories can tell us to purposely stop breathing until the sense of pain naturally tells us to follow our attractions and respire.

From the examples of the colored food, thirst and respiration, we see one of the great attributes of natural senses. They automatically blend and modify each other. In combination with the sense of reason, this enhances intelligent, thoughtful adaptability that promotes personal and global wholeness, even when our stories wrangle us not to do so. This is valuable in conflict resolution at all levels.

It is not intelligent for us to heed wranglers that disconnect our reasoning and stories from our natural senses. Disconnection reduces our ability to be reasonable, to think intelligently with respect to things like survival, clean air, healthy lungs, smoking, abusiveness, and overall wellness. Reconnecting with nature rejuvenates our natural senses and their wisdom. We bring our sense of self and integrity onto our consciousness screen. That is why it makes sense to reconnect, why it led Thoreau to say:

"Talk of mysteries! Think of our life in nature –daily to be shown matter, to come in contact with it–rocks, trees, wind on our cheeks! the solid earth! The actual world! the common sense! Contact! Contact! Who are we? Where are we?"

The Physiology of Nature-centered Thinking

Physiology researchers confirm that reconnecting with nature makes sense. They have established how the senses physiologically operate in us. For example, the intersensory communication in the colored food example takes place as thousands of cones and rods in the eye transform the food's color and shape into a group of electrical signals known as a nerve impulse. Simultaneously, the ears, nose, and skin. take in other data and transform it into electrical signals. Electrical signals from emotional responses (moods, pleasure, disapproval, etc.) combine with these signals to form a composite electrical message which is electrically and chemically transmitted to the brain along nerve cells and their connectors.

Radioisotope scans in the brain have shown that the signal travels between the mind's many perceptual regions like a ball in a pinball machine, including the areas of language and reason. Each region compares the signal to everything we have previously sensed. At phenomenal speed, electrical impulses and chemical substances bounce back and forth between these interconnected regions of the brain. They exchange signals, as well as store and retrieve them. A neurotransmitter then transports the modified signal out of the brain and back to its origins where it triggers appropriate behaviors.

The immensely accelerated neural process of our body-mind is almost a hologram of the process by which, over the eons, Earth's life community slowly and steadily communicates. Earth's neurons are the global flow of air, water, electric, magnetic, geologic, gravitational, and other attraction forces. We embody sensitivity to that process because each of our personal senses is a biological continuum of the global life community's interconnective properties and processes. In addition, evidence now suggests that on some level certain subatomic changes are universally known immediately. However, this hologram is only whole when it is connected to the whole. When connected to nature-separated paradigms, it produces a false image about our integrity on our screen of consciousness. Wholeness is not a story; it is being in attractive multisensory connection with the immediate environment. That's how nature works.

Nature's wisdom automatically heals areas disturbed by natural forces. Forest burns and tornado damage in time return to their former state. Nature in us also heals our scrapes, breaks, and bruises. Nature's multisensory intelligence knows how to heal and regenerate, how to keep us in balance. However, much of our upbringing wrangles us to trust and communicate through language stories that separate us from nature, not through stories that value making contact with nature's intelligence. Our social and environmental degradation show that we desperately need to create believable holistic stories, stories that reconnect us with the sensory global congress.

Although each natural sense participates in the natural world's governance, our nature-alienated indoor upbringing excessively emphasizes our consciousness of reasoning and language. These senses represent educational excellence, but they are only two of our many natural senses. They are part, but not all, of true wisdom. They are not our only way of knowing. Unlike ourselves, the global life community neither idolizes, restricts itself to, nor depends upon them alone. If rejuvenated and given the chance, the consensus of our congress of senses has the natural power to prevent our disconnected reasoning and language from continuing to mislead us.

The field of psychology often consists of studying and dealing with our separation from nature. It studies the effects of industrial society using stories to excessively separate us from our many other natural senses along with the rest of the natural world. Nature centered thinking and psychology goes a step further. It recognizes how words tend to mediate our natural sensations, hide them from our consciousness, and replace them with stories. In the process, we lose vital messages from nature itself. For example, whenever we let authorities wrangle us to conceptualize a natural area as so many square feet of economically valuable real estate, we tend to feel comfortable with thinking of it as an expendable exploitable object. It becomes a commodity or resource which we may bulldoze, clear-cut, develop, or otherwise capitalize on. This is different than personally gaining permission from a natural area to visit it and learn to know it from our multisensory experiences in it. Then our senses register the natural area on our screen of consciousness as much more. We may think of it as: an intimate part of ourselves, as a personal fulfillment, a friend, as love, as wisdom in action, a community, a home and life support system, a teacher, a biological necessity for one's ethical, physical and emotional well being, a celebration of billions of years of relating wisely, a spiritual or sacred place. Without our stories encouraging our consciousness to love a natural area because it is or possesses these qualities, we seldom treat natural areas or Earth with the respect they deserve. We do not do onto them as we would have others do onto us.

When we thoughtfully consider the list of 53 natural senses, we recognize that in congress these sensitivities govern the natural world and let us be conscious of the wholeness of nature. With the knowledge that these senses have a common origin in nature and are in our genetic code, it is reasonable to think that they make up a multisensory global mentality that we share with our planet. It is not a global brain, but rather it is a global intelligence, a way of being that manifests itself as Earth and can be found in some form in each member of the global life community. Of course, the sense that Earth is a multisensory intelligent being is foreign to our way of thinking. We have created and grown up in a people aggrandizing, nature-disconnected story that proves to be a limited-sense or nonsense (sic) way of thinking. Our story says that intelligence is humanity's ability to create stories that we can implement. In our civilization's present story, Earth's multisensory global intelligence and the people that use it are illiterate, uncivilized, and savage. The disastrous economics, misguided ethics, and severe mental and environmental distress of our civilization's story speak for themselves.

When we use people as an example of the effects of our stories, we must question our definition of intelligence. For example, when our nature-disconnected authorities teach us to conceptualize ourselves as having value, we learn to measure ourselves with respect to our cultural abilities to create and sustain our indoor world. We value our test scores, income, competitiveness, honors achieved, prestige, occupation, and language. We do not learn to pride ourselves as being our natural self, a knowledgeable participant in the global life community. That self is our dreams and fantasies, our yearnings for peace, fulfillment, joy, supportive community relationships, intimacy, natural beauty, sensibility, spirituality, trust, honesty, friendships, unity, and purity. Some of us assign these to heaven. These are also meaningful integrated directions for life on Earth! We learn to yearn for heaven as we learn to conquer and dehabilitate its fulfilling counterparts on Earth within and around us.

Thinking Like Nature: NIAL

By connecting with nature through consensual sensory contact with natural areas, we learn how to habitually think like nature works. We gravitate to what attracts us in a given moment. Our sense of reasoning makes our internal wranglers conscious that it is reasonable to trust nature's attributes. The intensity of your conviction about each of following four statements enables you to become aware of how strongly your sense of reason supports the nature reconnecting process at this time:

1) Nature is a nameless, nonverbal process.
2) Natural senses and nature are intelligent.
3) Natural senses in people are attractions to parts of nature.
4) Natural senses are forms of love that we feel.

The stronger your conviction, the greater your new brain readiness to voluntarily let Earth teach you to live in balanced sustainable simplicity with it.

The four attributes of nature connectedness listed above can be remembered by the acronym NIAL:

Namelessness: non-language ways of relating, knowing and feeling.

Intelligence: the natural ability for attractions to blend in supportive ways

Attractions: natural energies that draw things together.

Love: Our ability to enjoyably feel nature's attraction process

We think with nature when we are in conscious contact with NIAL within or around us. It is part of natural love that we can easily experience and validate by reconnecting with nature. Connection with NIAL always feels good because it brings to consciousness the ability of natural attractions to balance themselves. For example, planet Earth stays on its course around the sun because it lies in balance between its gravitational attractions to the Sun and its centerfugal and other forces to move into space. On some level, this is the process that every entity in nature experiences, be they animal, vegetable, or mineral.

When we think in ways that exclude NIAL, we end up with stories and relationships that continuously conflict with each other. These stories often lead us to a stressed state of being. Without NIAL, we think our way into destructive perceptions and problems of race, nationality, sex, religion, and economics. Nature's intelligence in us avoids these problems. We have lost this ability due to our estrangement from nature. It has lead us to DE-NIAL!

The stories told by nature-centered societies enable them to enjoy NIAL, the dream of Earth that they genetically and culturally inherit. They disavow the fantasy of nature conquest that predicates our existence. Our troubles emanate from wrangling, subdividing, alienating, or killing our natural desire to be connected to nature. We regain wholeness by getting out of deNIAL, by reconnecting and letting nature help sustain multisensory contact and balance.

Activity 6: Learning From Sensory Nature Connecting

Go to an attractive natural area. As you did in the previous activities, ask for the natural area's permission for you to become involved with it. Gain its consent and thank it for helping you with this activity.

The words psyche and spirit are ancient names for air. Green plants naturally produce oxygen, the part of air we breathe that sustains our lives. Air is a product of nature. So is our sensory desire to breathe. We call the process respiration, meaning *re-spiriting*.

Approach a green plant in this area and have your conscious mind tell yourself to "stop breathing." Then actually stop breathing as your verbal command has requested. This disconnects an important part of you from nature. Notice the disruptive natural feeling of suffocation that comes into play and intelligently asks you to reconnect by breathing again. That feeling or sensation is one of your 53 natural senses in action. It is making sense.

Only allow yourself to start breathing again by holding onto, or embracing, part of the plant because it produces the oxygen you need for survival. This lets your natural senses feelingly bring to your new brain an awareness that the plant supports you. Notice the rewarding natural feeling that comes into play when you breathe again. It comes from the fulfillment of your natural sense of respiration. Release the plant, stop breathing again for as long as you want, and repeat the whole process. Do this for 15 minutes or more. Note what changes, if any, occur from doing this activity. What happens if you do this activity but hold an artifact like an air freshener, deodorant, or air-conditioner instead of a plant? Does holding them feel the same as holding the plant? Does the word "respiration" have different meaning now?

Recognize that each time you exhale, the carbon dioxide in your breath feeds the green part of a plant.

Write down the three most important things you learned from this chapter and activity.

Write down what good feelings/sensations were brought on when you held the plant and resumed breathing.

How would you feel about giving up the ability to have those feelings?

Does this activity enhance your sense of self-worth?

Chapter Seven

Replenishing Earth and its People:
The RWN Factor

Letting nature recharge our battery of 53 natural senses brings balance to our personal and collective lives.

In recent times idealism has become a dirty word. Perhaps it is because our runaway social and environmental deterioration tramples our ideals. We seem helpless to stop the juggernaut, so instead of ideals, we seek practical solutions, things that work. I suggest that a practical solution is to use proven nature-connecting activities to replenish our deficiency of natural attraction sensations. Only when we replenish our love of, by, and from nature will the deterioration halt. Lest this sound idealistic, consider the following incident. It addresses the ingrained ways of a supposedly unchangeable group of hard core killers:

In the West Virginia mountains, an isolated, dedicated hunting club finds a month old male fawn whose mother has been killed by a car. For a week, these middle aged men, each with decades of devoted deer killing expertise, decide to feed the fawn formula from a bottle, which it suckles with half shut eyes of ecstasy. In return the fawn licks their hands, sucks their earlobes and sings them little whining sounds of delight from deep within. When the hunt breaks up, these men disperse leaving the fawn eating grass and craving its bottle. They make vague promises to return to this remote place. Individually, as time permits, they trek to the mountain and feed the fawn. A few weeks later, one of the hunters phones the others to see if anybody knows if the fawn has been fed or has survived. He discovers that without each other knowing it, five of the hunters often visit the fawn and feed it, so it is actually getting fat. Although the fawn might be shot by someone who did not know the situation, it lifts his heart to think that the fawn has a chance at life because some hardened deer hunters have gone out of their way to care for him. He knows for sure that none of his hunt club members would shoot this deer.

It is worth noting in this true-life experience that neither a teacher nor a preacher appeared to educate the hunters about the value of the fawn's life. Although it said not a word, the fawn was the educator. The beauty and integrity of its life touched the lives of the hunters. The connection sparked into consciousness their inherent attraction feelings of love. NIAL expressed itself as many natural senses: nurturing, empathy, community, friendship, power, humility, reasoning, and a score of others. Reconnecting moments with nature rejuvenated a battery of different natural senses. These new feelings led a group of deer hunters to support rather than deny the life of a deer and bring joy to their personal and collective lives. Was there not at least a touch of this nature supportive feeling in your personal nature experience that you recounted in chapter 1? Did you find traces of this feeling in the activities of the past chapters? Do you trust this feeling?

Remember that all of this emanated from but one contact with one aspect of nature. What I have found is the means by which any person can choose to have many such moments daily with many aspects of nature in the environment, people, and themselves. Each moment feels good, uplifting, and responsible. These moments are like lollipops of life. In a relatively short time they create a habitual way of thinking and relating that reverses the deterioration in ourselves and the environment. I suggest that such moments are a reconnecting-with-nature (RWN) factor whose absence from our personal lives produces our unsolvable personal and global problems.

Although the daily insertion of an RWN factor into our nature-separated lives sounds ideal, it is within the grasp of any individual that knows of its existence. It is now a tested and proven vehicle to mental and environmental health, a responsible way of thinking and acting that most people learn in less than six months. It is also the core of societies that do not suffer from our problems. I conservatively estimate that at least 600 million people in industrial society alone can learn to integrate and enjoy the RWN factor at home, work, and school. As people learn it, they can teach it formally. Even if they don't teach it, they inject it into their personal and professional relationships because it provides immediate rewards for them, their community, and the environment. In that way, others learn RWN from them.

The following question is so important that I will repeat it many times throughout this book: What would our world be like if 600 million people had RWN experiences daily? What if these experiences triggered unifying senses, feelings, and acts similar to those of the deer hunters and the fawn?

That thought is the essence of the RWN factor and that thought is not ours alone. In some form that thought is shared by the nature of every member of the global life community, no matter their cultural differences or species. The sense in that thought is the love of life, an essence of the fawn, the hunter and life itself. It is a natural, unifying intelligence.

Activity 7: Unity With Nature

Part One:

Let nature help you discover the unity and community you share. Go to an attractive natural area. As you did in the previous activities, ask for the natural area's permission for you to visit and become involved with it. Gain its consent to help you with this activity.

For one minute simply walk through that natural community. For the next minute continue to walk through it while repeating the word "unity" over and over again. Think about the many interrelationships of the community that surrounds you. Repeat this process for 10 minutes. See what differences, if any, you observe when you think "unity" as opposed to when you don't.

Write down the three most important things you learned from this activity.

Write down what, if any, good feelings were brought on by doing this activity. Can you describe them?

Part Two:

Think about a person you respect or love.

What qualities do they have that make them attractive to you?

Is this person abnormal or do most people have these attractive natural qualities somewhere within them?

If you appreciate these qualities, it means that part of you is sensitive to and aware of them. That part of you is that quality in you. You were born with it. It is part of your nature that, unnurtured, has not yet fully expressed itself. Chances are, that quality is naturally found in most people and throughout nature. Our nature- disconnected society seldom nurtures it effectively. Note that these attraction qualities are also found in other species, they are not ours alone. They are the natural qualities, held in common, that sustain the Earth community. They are the "unity" in global community.

Write down the three most important things you learned from this activity. Write down what, if any, good feelings were brought on by doing this activity. Can you describe them? How would you feel about giving up the ability to have those feelings or if the ability to feel them was taken away? Does this activity enhance your sense of self-worth?

Chapter Eight

Reconnecting With Nature

To habitually think in multisensory ways is to consistently be inspired by nature's beauty within us.

My 35 exploratory years in nature have shown me a major cause of today's runaway degradation of people and places. Our most challenging problems result from the difference between nature's ways and the nature-separated thinking of our industrial society. Our education, formal and informal, teaches us to pay attention to the stressful complexities of managing life through stories about life rather than to participate in it. Our ill effects suggest that the global life experience itself has enough sense(s) to know how to manage itself far better than we do. However, we can reconnect with global life and learn how to let it show us what we need to know.

At birth, every human being is born as part of nature itself. Like nature itself, an infant is born out of love, not fear. Fear of people and nature is absent in the newborn. In addition, nature does not teach an infant to destroy natural areas or to create garbage, war, or insanity. These learnings are not originally part of the human soul. Our civilization, our process of becoming civilized, teaches these things to us.

Any intelligent civilization's mandate, as in all of nature, is to gain consent from nature to survive. Any form of life's mandate is to organize itself to nurture nature's supportive ways within and around it. The civilizing process has never gained permission to abuse the natural person or the environment. To assault nature is to go against nature's wisdom, to create unnatural problems with destructive effects. That is a lesson we have learned all too well. Reconnecting with nature reverses our destructive processes. It creates tangible connections with nature and an environmentally responsible psychology that enables us to unlearn our destructive personal, social, and environmental ways.

Increasingly, we face frightening relationships. Our society produces them every time it teaches us to believe we may live and think in excessive separation from nature. Although Earth's nurturing life process is an essence of our soul and survival, society teaches us that we may learn to think rationally and survive happily while isolated from nature/Earth . The negative effects of doing this explicitly say otherwise. Like a contagious disease, our nature-separated thoughts and ways initiate much of the runaway destruction we find across the face of our planet.

Some Indian friends of mine tell me they are proud to be called Indians. They say that diaries written by Columbus show that he called some tribes of their people "Indians" not because he thought he was in India, but because he observed that these hunter/gatherer tribes happily lived with nature and God, "En Dios." Thus, they clain that "En Dios" is the origin of "Indians." Further support of this claim is that India was not even called India in 1492. Some, but by no means all, ancient natural tribal communities embraced a psychology that identified spirit and nature as a singular relationship. The effects of them doing this deserves our attention. These nature-connected people knew how to live harmoniously with each other and the land. Some did so for over 50 thousand years. Their psychology helped balance person, nature, and spirit. Today, through the methods and materials this book offers, any person can apply that psychology to modern life and benefit themselves and Earth.

Living in integrity creates lasting satisfaction. As we learn to separate from nature, we lose our natural integrity and its blessings. Most individuals, families, or communities that sustain a semblance of lasting happiness today are those that painstakingly choose to reconnect themselves with nature's ways and wisdom. Happiness achieved otherwise is usually a short-term affair. It is a tranquilizer, a delusion that hides from consciousness the discomfort from our confinement within our society's intellectual walls and adverse effects. Too often, our civilized walls protect us from contacting and feeling first hand the pain of our hurtful effects. In this way, the walls encourage us to dance on the deck of our sinking ship rather than stop the leaks. Nature within and around us abhors the vacuum our walls create. Nature cries for help by creating the pain and disorders of today's world and our lives. That pain demands that we do something more attractive, more responsible

Most members of the education, mental health, and political communities have yet to recognize that our personal, social, and environmental problems have a common cause: our excessive separation from nature. They do not know how nature works in sensory ways.

Sadly, greed still blinds many us from believing that a planetary survival problem even exists. John Dewey and many others have observed that we do not begin to think until we are confronted with a problem. Without even admitting our problems and without effective methods to change our present course, we have little cause for hope. Unfortunately, many of society's deep misguided ideas die only as those that hold them die. Even when a bloody revolution occurs, too often what remains is faith in the process of bloody revolution. That is not nature's way.

Our excessive separation from nature holds each of us hostage. We neither see nor validate nature's magnificent process of peaceful, natural change. That process offers a revolutionary but peaceful solution. It is the process by which nature sustains an optimum of life, diversity and beauty without producing our runaway pollution, war, or violence. It offers things that work, things we can do.

We should trust and learn from thoughtful and rewarding experiences with nature. For example:

In Scotland, farmers overturn their hay bales to exterminate rats that live beneath them. A trio of rats tries to flee but, unlike the other fleeing rats, these three stay closely together which limits their ability to escape. This attracts the farmers. Upon investigation, they find that the middle rat of the three is blind; its companions are guiding it to safety. Deeply moved, the farmers do not kill these rats. Instead, in awe, they respect them.

We often call the farmers' response "human morality, values, ethics," or "being humane." However, these words hide that even rats, through their natural attractions, "morally" respond in the same way as did the farmers, and rats have done so for millions of years before humanity came into being. Similar animal and plant behavior is common throughout the natural world. For example, the beautiful intricate patterns that colonies of bacteria form, or the shape of a coral reef result from how individual organisms in these communities communicate with each other and disseminate information throughout the colony. The behavior of these earliest forms of life show that they change their behavior in response to changing environmental conditions, not through random genetic mutation. To survive, they cooperatively signal, calculate, network, regulate and control their community behavior in response to environmental conditions. The patterns they produce are the same as those found in minerals, suggesting that the same process exists on molecular and atomic levels. Genetically, the same process enables lactose intolerant bacteria to become lactose tolerant and thereby survive. However, our mentality's disconnection from nature prevents us from saying the farmers acted naturally, like rats, bacteria or other species.

The farmers, rats, and microorganisms clearly demonstrate that nature connecting experiences can teach us what our society's story about nature can't. Think again about what our world would be like if 600 million people had daily RWN experiences with nature and their community, experiences similar to those of the farmers and the three rats. That thought is the essence of the RWN factor and that thought is not ours alone. In some form that thought is shared by every member of the global life community, no matter their cultural differences or species. The sense in that thought is the love of life, an essence of the farmers, rats, microorganisms, and life itself.

Activity 8: Separation from nature

Industrial society lives by a story that guides us to separate from nature and our natural senses. Discover the effects of this story. Go to an attractive natural area. As you did in the previous activities, ask for the natural area's permission for you to become involved with it. Gain its consent to help you with this activity.

Wrap a towel or sweater around one of your hands. Now shut your eyes. With your eyes closed, carefully, gently feel natural things in the immediate area with both your wrapped and unwrapped hand. Repeat this procedure with your eyes open.

Write what you sense, think, and feel from this experience. Try to make sense of it. This activity asks your new brain to consciously experience sensory disconnection from nature.

Some past participant's reactions may be of help. The last one is especially significant:

"The covered hand was warmer and more protected, but it seldom felt the outside world and it wanted to. It was frustrated. It sensed things differently than did the bare hand. It was comparatively numb and uninteresting."

"The wrapped hand saddened me, but thinking about what having to wear the wrapping meant in terms of my natural attractions and my overprotected, indoor childhood frustrated me. I got angry."

"Nothing is anybody's fault. Our society's stories threaten our inner child when they tell us to wear the wrapping or be abandoned."

"The damn wrapping is a lie that we're forced to learn. The thicker the wrapping, the less I could sense or make sense."

"This activity helps me see how sensory numbness results from a person living excessively indoors. It explains how people can become insensitive. I had to bang on things in order to feel them with the covered hand. My insensitivity changed my impact, how I felt I had to relate."

Write down the three most important things you learned from this activity.

Write down what good feelings were brought on by doing this activity.

If it taught you something worthwhile, does that feel good? Can you describe the feeling?

How would you feel about giving up the ability to have that feeling?

Does this activity enhance your natural sense of self-worth?

Chapter Nine

People and Nature as Community

Over the eons, nature's multisensory intelligence has increased life's diversity and itself.

Our natural self is like a sensory Velcro®. It sustains itself by seeking, loving, and attaching to every physical, mental, and spiritual support available in natural people and places. These supports become its sensory community.

Our indoor life does not have what our natural self usually needs to be nurtured, safe, and satisfied. For example: although she sits comfortably in a modern temperature controlled room in downtown Seattle, Brenda feels unsafe. She is a participant in one of my reconnecting with nature classes, a practicing 31 year old mental health worker, a graduate student, and mother of two. She, along with many of her colleagues, have decided to be honest with each other and have ended up anxious and hurt. Like most people I know, they think the world has gone crazy and part of themselves went with it.

As we look at our lives and all of life, we realize that people and nature are being brutalized. Although most of us deeply feel it is wrong, we don't know how to stop it on global or personal levels. Many say they want to feel closer to each other and themselves. They want to be in a community, to build supportive immediate relationships that they can trust. However, they can't converse easily and they don't feel safe with each other, even though some are members of the same family. This upsets Brenda. Softly crying, Brenda says: "I hate community, I hate trying to build closer relationships. They always become tense and stressful like this. My inner nature would much rather live alone than put up with the discomfort and bewilderment I feel right now. I'm confused because, although I feel hurt, nobody is actually hurting me. Actually, every person here and every other sensitive person I know or work with wants to be in community. So why am I upset, what's going on?" Overwhelmed, she pauses for a moment, then sobs: "And why do I have to lie to you? Why can't I honestly tell you that I actually long for warm connections with you and others, with people I trust. It must be natural...I have wanted to give and receive trust and love as long as I can remember.... why should that be so hard, so risky and painful?" She pauses again, wipes her tears, and asks: "Why should I have to suffer to fulfill my desire for closeness? Why, as an adult, am I still such a child as to still want supportive relationships....what's wrong with me.....or them....why can't I grow up? I'm an adult. I'm successful, doing well at something I like and is useful, so why does it hurt? I feel like three entirely different people in the same body: one wants to live responsibly in a supportive community, another fears it, and a third is so hardened to the idea that it thinks the whole idea is idealistic and ridicules the other two parts of me for being immature."

Brenda is at odds with herself because neither she nor our society are whole with respect to Earth and how nature works. She is conflicted. The story she has learned about who she should be is at odds with who she naturally is. Brenda and every other living being depend upon their environment to support their being. We each consist of many desires for consent for our life to be. Without this consent, our life ceases. Whenever full consent is not present, we cannot achieve our full potential. Consent nourishes and supports the roots for individuality and cooperation. A wholesome person is the product of a wholesome environment, of surroundings that support the individual's innate desire to relate and grow.

Brenda's sadness and conflicts touch each of us in the room. They strike feelings we hold and bring them into our awareness again. A profound silence prevails, finally broken by Roberta. "I'd like to talk about what we each feel right now," she says and she begins to emote her frustrations.

"Roberta, may I interrupt for a moment?" I ask. "Can we take a moment to see if we all agree that this is what we want to do?"

Roberta consents but, frustrated, Bill and then Sarah question my suggestion. "Why we must agree to do it when she is already doing it?" they ask.

I respond, "In today's disconnected world, close relationships best form when we make a safe space for them to happen. We must learn to consciously, thoughtfully, consent to relate sensibly and to support each other as we do it. That makes it safe to for us to relate in wholeness, in ways that include everybody and that include nature."

"But, what's wrong with just doing it?" asks Bob.

"Without consenting to connect with nature and share our feelings," I reply, "we don't start off practicing the safe community process we want to master. Giving our consent to make it happen lets us purposely build and enter a sanctuary. The sanctuary, in turn, enables us to reasonably and safely risk learning how to sustain and extend it. Without sensibly consenting to the process, the mistrust that ordinarily surrounds and embodies us remains, it prevents community from forming. Does that make sense?"

"I get it," says Bob, "if we don't consciously consent to make it happen, we are not in charge of it being safe, so how can we trust that it is safe? Okay, Roberta has made a splendid suggestion. I commit to supporting it. How do others feel?"

Without dissent, the group agrees to openly and honestly share their thoughts and feelings about reconnecting with nature and each other. In the 30 minutes that follow, frustrations, disappointments, and hopes for each other and Earth pour out in relative safety. Each participant takes the risk of expressing their inborn natural love of community with others and Earth, for each knows they have gained support to do so. Each recognizes, on some level, that, unlike times in their past, they will not be rejected or "punished" for being who they really are. Although one woman finds that doing this triggers too many painful past experiences and opts to leave temporarily, the rest of us feel more attracted to her, each other, and this natural community process. Even though each of us are still uncomfortable, our discomfort is something we hold in common and share so we also feel more supported and more alive in this challenging setting and moment. We are rationally learning to deal with our reality, our lives, and life on Earth. Why the discomfort? Because we are doing it indoors. What is missing is the safety, support, and nurturing that natural attractions in natural areas provide all species including humanity. That sanctuary was made and consists of a wisdom greater than our own whose loss has proven to be a missing link in the way we think. The dire effects of its absence speak for themselves personally and globally. A week later when the same class met in a natural area and did reconnective activities, the stress between them became support that nurtured them.

My indoor classes in Seattle are not where I usually teach. For over three decades I have lived and taught in close-knit group settings in natural areas. Some groups met over a period of many years. Participants ranged from 15 to 50 years old, single to married, and included many different ethnicities, occupations, and lifestyles.

In the natural areas my trailside program visited, we learned from nature how to let our inborn love of life help us supportively relate to each other and the environment. For this reason, during our scheduled vacation periods, participants and staff seldom wanted to go home. Why should we want to leave? Our attractive connections with nature enabled us to build a community that felt more sensible and worthwhile than anything we had previously experienced, often including our families. Outfitted only with a vehicle, camping gear, and a small library, we spent the year sleeping out under storms and bright stars throughout the seasons; camping, exploring and learning in nature's beauty. The consensus-governed outdoor-living Trailside program that I founded in 1959 immersed itself in critical thinking, rich multisensory experiences, and nature's magnificence. Participants thrived in 83 different natural habitats! In keeping their commitments to open, honest relationships with the natural environment and each other, participants including researchers, ecologists, Amish farmers, anthropologists, folk musicians, naturalists, shamans, administrators, historians and many others built lasting relationships. The process deeply connected our inner nature to the whole of nature. In 1977, *The New York Times* said the program was: "A pioneer in the environmental education movement. Participants learn to learn, they learn that all subjects are interrelated with one another and themselves. Most of all, they develop an interest in themselves." Robert Binnewies, Vice President of the National Audubon Society called Trailside: "the most revolutionary school in America."

As a result of educating ourselves in this nature reconnected way:

Chemical dependencies, including alcohol and tobacco, disappeared as did destructive social relationships.

Personality and eating disorders subsided.

Violence, crime and prejudice were unknown in the group.

Loneliness, hostility and depression subsided. Group interactions allowed for stress release and management; each day was fulfilling and relatively peaceful.

Students using meditation found they no longer needed to use it to feel fulfilled.

Participants knew each other better than they knew their families or best friends.

Participants risked expressing and acting from their deeper thoughts and feelings; a profound sense of social and environmental responsibility and support guided their decisions.

When vacation periods arrived, nobody wanted to go home. Each person enjoyably worked hard to build this supportive, balanced living and learning utopia. They were home.

All this occurred simply because every community member met their commitment to make sense of their lives by establishing attractive relationships that supported the natural world within and around them. We hunted, gathered, and practiced such relationships; we organized and preserved group living processes that awakened our natural wisdom. We learned to regenerate responsible relationships when they decayed. The secret to our success was to learn how to learn directly from the natural world, the living earth within and about us. Through our natural sensations and feelings nature taught us how to trust it, how to validate and incorporate life experience.

From 30 years of all-season travel and study in over 260 national parks, forests, and subcultures, I developed a repeatable learning process and psychology that unleashes our natural attraction ability to grow and survive responsibly. By documenting that it works repeatedly and can be taught, I earned a doctoral degree and the school became a small graduate and undergraduate degree program.

To share my discovery with the public, I encapsulated my nature reconnecting process in a series of 107 published sensory activities in 1988. People do them in their backyard, a park, or back country, and achieve the same results I obtained at the Trailside program. Today, on the Internet, I use these activities to teach counselors, educators, and other participants worldwide how to incorporate them into their lives. The program benefits people of all ages and backgrounds. As it revitalizes natural sensory communication, it connects our consciousness with its origins–the natural wisdom, joy, and beauty found in ourselves, others, and natural areas.

Some Native American people tell me that my nature reconnecting activities simulate how many Indians learn from the Great Circle of Life to live in harmony with it, and how they miss doing that in their modern lives. What they say brings to my mind the year of 1983 when my students and I were privileged to attend Kachina night dances in a small northern Arizona Indian village. The next day we sat with Maria, an old Hopi grandmother wedged in her tiny living room below the pueblo. We listened intently to her story.

"They wanted us to learn their white ways," Maria said. They brought in the U.S. Army to make us go to school." Her voice was soft as she stared at the floor and remembered her childhood. "But still my parents and other Hopis resisted. The soldiers, every morning they came with guns, went from house to house, searching for children–so every morning, very early, one of my people would gather us children away to hide..." She gave a strained laugh.

American society traditionally has viewed the Native American as an anomaly. They are thought of as a nature connected race of savages, not quite human; a feral and cunning people living in primitive conditions, close to nature. We have, in the same tradition, done our best to change that. Our society's past includes a holocaust that proclaimed: "The only good Indian is a dead Indian." We taught the Indians that survived to learn and live the ways of our nature- isolated lives.

"One by one we were found and caught," continued Maria. "Children and parents would be crying; the soldier would have one of your arms, your mother the other; and you were pulled away, kicking, from everything you naturally know, to go to the Indian school in Phoenix. You did not come home again for twelve years. I was one of those children," she said, and she gave a nervous, high pitched laugh. They were Indian children, angels of Satan, the uncivilized children of nature that we forcibly educated to our ways.

"We did not have our lessons in Hopi; they were in English. Hopi was forbidden. We did not understand English, but we were punished if we were heard speaking Hopi amongst ourselves. We could not be who we were." She laughed nervously. "The principal had a pistol full of blank cartridges. He used to fire it over the heads of the bigger boys to frighten them into obeying the rules. The food was strange to us, but if we did not eat what we were served, we went hungry. We were not allowed to go home in the summer for fear that perhaps we would not come back–so we were put to work at summer jobs. Anyway, after a few years we would not fit in at home. We were changed," she tittered.

The living room was taut with an amazed silence, broken only by the nervous laugh with which Maria punctuated every statement. She showed no resentment for the treatment she and other Hopi children had received. The only sign of her discomfort was her recurring, apologetic laugh, as she looked up from the floor and read the horror in our eyes that reflected some long-ignored part of herself.

We remembered the Hopi schoolteacher who the previous day told us, "American education is the weapon that has finally invaded and conquered the formerly invincible Hopi, a peaceful natural people who once successfully repelled both Coronado and Christianity." Now we understood.

Maria gestured around the room at the three television sets, the stereo, the bookcases full of books, the couch, the electric drier, the coffee table, the wall-to-wall carpet. "Now I am an American," she said proudly. But there was a deep crease between her brows and she tittered.

To this day, remembering Maria's nervous laugh disturbs me. It reminds me of the inadequacy of the psychology that professionals used to heal the hurt from her separation from her natural community origins. She still feels it, she knows it is there. The best healing of her inner pain might have been to let her return home and contribute to productive family and community life. It was there that she was wanted, loved, and nurtured and where she wanted to be. Today, she lives as an outsider of her traditional Hopi community. She typifies the lives of many of the relocated Hopi children. They are disillusioned and often exploited by industrial society. They return home even though they feel somewhat isolated from those who were not removed. They return because their natural community ways make more sense to them and feel more supportive.

The separation of Hopi young people from their natural social community is relevant to our lives because Western Civilization has also torn most of us and our natural attractions from our attractions, roots, and home in nature and community. Although spiritual questions may arise with respect to our deep relationship with the natural world, biologically, no question exists. We are rooted in nature, we are to nature as our leg is to our body. Not only do my many years living in natural areas allow me to feel this deep connection, many impeccable sources of information constantly validate it.

It is no accident that the word human has its ancient roots in humus, a fertile forest soil. One teaspoon of humus consists of water, minerals and many other species. Each one contains about five million bacteria, twenty million fungi, one million protozoa and two hundred thousand algae, all living cooperatively in an integrity that supports life. This coincides with our bodies containing water, minerals, and ten times as many cells of nonhuman species as human cells. We are as humus. Over half our body weight consists of the weight of "foreign" microorganism species; over 115 different species live on our skin alone. We and nature are so close that some microorganisms have complete life cycles within each human cell, cycles that integrate with and support each cell's life. Remove or kill these microorganisms and the human cell dies. Similar microorganisms not only embody us, but every other form of life as well.

Biologists and chemists demonstrate that the natural world constantly flows around and through us. They show that every 5-7 years every molecule in our body is continually replaced, particle by particle, by new molecules attracted in from the environment and vice-versa. The natural environment becomes our body and we become it a dozen or more times during our lifetime. We and nature are each other.

Earth is a cohesive life system of which we are part. It nurtures us and we it. To be part of any system, we must in some way be in contact with the system. Disconnected parts often go their separate ways or violate the system unwittingly. This means that since we are part of the natural system, nature must communicate with us in some way. We learn to ignore that communication, so it seems invisible to us. We rarely identify or validate how nature communicates with us, yet it does so continuously.

Even people without scientific training recognize that everything in nature is connected, everything attracts or attaches to something else. We know that the global life system holds itself together through a variety of affinity attractions. It communicates through these natural attractions. From atomic nuclei to matter to weather systems, attractions interact, connect, form, and sustain nature, including us. The space within each atom is not empty, it is filled with attractions that hold the atom together. They blast fiery nuclear anger when forcibly separated to produce atomic explosions along with lasting radioactive pollution. Both are ordinarily unknown on Earth.

We register and may become conscious of nature's attraction energies. They register as our natural sensations and feelings: senses like thirst, hunger, beauty, nurturing, taste, smell, and the like. We sometimes call these survival senses loves, faculties, or instincts.

Together, we and nature are an interconnected intelligent integrity. Every person shares one breath with all species and life systems. Emerson and many others noted that everything in nature is made of one hidden stuff. Each thing contains all the powers of nature when nurtured by nature's cohesiveness. For example, when people of our culture marry aboriginal people, the children are healthy and fertile. Biologically, we and the aboriginal are one. This means that each of us carry within us genetically the inherent natural attraction wisdom and integrity of aboriginal people. They are a people who, in conjunction with nature, have used this wisdom to live in harmony with the land and each other for multiple thousands of years.

In their questioning and sadness, some participants in my workshops and courses first come to recognize the depth of what has happened to them as members of our industrial society. With respect to being disconnected from nature and natural community, they have much in common with the Hopi youngsters that were disconnected from their tribal community's supportive nature-loving ways. The authorities in our modern lives –parents, educators, presidents– teach us to spend an average of over 95% of our life indoors. For example, we are "sentenced" to spending over 18,000 hours of our developmental childhood years indoors in classrooms or else suffer the pains of truancy. That makes our indoor schooling a mind- possessing subculture as well as educational. This statement may seem extreme, but as I write another bill is before the legislature authorizing jail sentences for truant students.

Learning to tolerate excessive existence indoors is as much a part of our education as are books, videos, and lectures. We have already achieved excellence in this aspect of our education. We educate ourselves with indoor thinking, media, and responsibilities to the extent that we average less than one day per lifetime in sensory tune with the natural world. If we look at ourselves and our society objectively, we observe ourselves to be a closeted, crippled people, traumatically torn from the integrity of nature and culturally blocked from reconnecting with it. Most of us sense this loss, this sensory sterility. Psychologist Raymond Sierra says: "People are an integral part of nature. As we learn to assault the natural world around us, we learn to assault our true inner nature, and vice versa." The hurt from this assault fuels our disorders.

Sadly, the despair and the lack of supportive community that too many of us feel is common throughout America. It results from our separation from nature. Most people are aware of this on some level. They know that when we genuinely reconnect with nature, our stressed feelings wane. However, they usually reappear when we return home from our outings.

Although we may intellectually give credence to the rationality of being with nature, most of our lives consist of physical and emotional disconnection from our natural origins. Although we may deny it, our daily life assaults and displaces nature's essence in our soul and spirit, just as it does in the environment. We have learned thinking and skills that support cement school buildings, asphalt parking lots and economic relationships. We demand that huge amounts of time be spent in that environment. An immense, beautiful, natural essence of ourselves feels dead. Its absence hurts.

Our incredible bewilderment (wilderness separation) blinds us from seeing that our many personal and global problems primarily result from our assault of and separation from the natural creation process within and around us. Our estrangement from nature leaves us wanting, and when we want there is never enough. Our insatiable wanting is called greed. It is a major source of our destructive dependencies and violence. When I authentically rejoin people with nature, they want less. They also get smarter about not letting themselves get hurt. Then problems dissolve. *The New York Times* understated it when an article observed that communion with Earth sharpens the insight. This is now being noted by psychotherapists, as it was earlier by Thoreau.

Throughout Western history and thought, many people have observed the value of reconnecting with nature. It is not some trendy psychology. It is the act of going home to nature, our biological home, and feeling nurtured. We reconnect to life's innate happiness by removing the walls that restrain us from dancing with it. The psychology of the process consists of finding language to scientifically explain why it works. Sadly, if our society wasn't so excessively separated from nature, there would be a lot less need for psychological studies and therapies. We mostly need psychology to heal the rift with nature that we have been trained to choose to live in. That's why today's growing field of ecopsychology abounds with psychotherapists and researchers who validate the nature-reconnecting process in some form. Wendall Berry and many others suggest that we hold Earth in common; what we do to it, we do to ourselves.

The idea of reconnecting with nature is nothing new. Zeno expressed it in 520 BC when he said: "The purpose of life is to live in agreement with nature." Our common culture continually chooses to ignore that ancient statement and heed instead the great American nature-separated dream. What is new is that sensory nature reconnecting activities enable people to live, at will, in attractive agreement with nature and their inner nature. The activities offer us a simple choice: reconnect with nature or live with the dire consequences of feeling and being disconnected from deeper wisdom and joys of life.

Earth and its people are stressed and at risk. By learning how to reconnect with nature we may tangibly participate in nature's ways and reap important insights and rewards. Consider what ecopsychologists have discovered about reconnecting with nature, as reported by *The New York*

Times in 1993:

"On wilderness trips many or most people undergo profound changes in their personal relationships or in the direction for their life's work. They report an increased awakeness and power, a sense of energies obtained from nature." -Robert Greenway

"In nature, there was a definite perspective shift. It quickly downsizes your preoccupation with problems in you career or private world." -Tim Gillen

"The individualism emphasized by American psychology and culture separates us from one another and from Earth itself. That leaves us feeling alone and helpless when confronted with the Earth's distress. Then our recourse is to deny our connection, to numb our senses and to continue our destructive assault." -Sarah Conn

"There is an ecological unconscious that can be drawn on to restore people to harmony with the natural world, a bond between our species and the planet as tenacious as the sexual instincts Freud found in the psyche." -Theodore Roszak

What I and others have found effective in my nature reconnecting work has long been known. St. Augustine observed it 1,600 years ago suggesting that it is how little we know of nature that makes nature seem like a miracle. If we want nature's wisdom and miracles to assist our personal lives and life on Earth, it makes sense to consciously make let tangible affirming contacts with nature to awaken nature's miraculous creativity and wisdom that lies within us. "Speak to the Earth and it shall teach thee," says Job 12:8. Theodore Roszak offers that Sigmund Freud explained it when he said: "A man who is in love declares that I and You are one and is prepared to behave as if it were a fact." When our thinking includes our love for nature and Earth, it includes the wholeness, balance, and wisdom of our biological Earth mother. The chapters that follow scientifically show you the how and why needed to creatively engage in the art of nature connected thinking and relating. Their effects are conveyed in the following example:

In Maine, a tough wildlife warden who enforces the Marine Mammals Protection Act inspects a wildlife rehabilitation center that nurses abandoned seal pups to health and then releases them. Nothing is more captivating than a baby seal. Their pleading inquisitive eyes and playful ways naturally charm most people. However, fishermen accuse seals of decimating fish populations, so seal protection contains certain limits. The law allows only seal pups that are abandoned because of proven adverse human activity to be rehabilitated. If unproven, all other abandoned pups are left to die. The warden and the director of the rehab center visit a beach. They discover an abandoned seal pup that is caught under a rock. They free it and the warden, upon asking, is told that if left on its own, the seal pup will die. Under the natural attractions spell of the pup, the warden somehow finds a way to allow it to be rehabilitated even though human intervention has not been proven. Ten weeks later the seal pup is released in good health.

Again, think about what the global community would be like if 600 million people in it had daily reconnecting with nature experiences including those similar to the director, the warden, and the seal. Those experiences are available and they produce a global consciousness we sorely need. They are the essence of the RWN factor. Every member of the global life community shares that consciousness, no matter their culture or species. The sense in that awareness is the love of life, an essence of the warden, the seal, and life itself.

Activity 9: Discovering Our Natural Self

This is a two-part reconnecting activity you can do to help your new brain validate your connections to the global life community in and around you.

PART 1:

Go to an attractive plant, animal, mineral, or place in a natural area. Thankfully ask for its permission to become involved with it. Gain its consent to help you with this activity. Do the following activity once you are sure the natural thing you selected continues to give you some sort of comfortable, attractive feeling. Be sure that you like this natural attraction.

Write down what you like and why. This may be as simple as: The plant, animal, mineral, place or thing in this natural area that I like is (1) _____. I like it because (2)_____ (Complete this sentence fully. State why you like the natural thing you chose and entered in (1). This is a NIAL centered statement.

PART 2:

Be sure you have completed part 1.
Note: This activity will not be helpful if what you liked in nature is a hurtful aspect of nature rather than a comfortable one
Instructions:
Place the phrase "I like myself because" in front of your "why" sentence from part 1 and the "because it" clause of the sentence. Now read the sentence including the new prefix: "I like myself because" sentence aloud. Read it to others, if possible. How does the whole sentence feel? Does it describe part of you? For example: "I like the tree because it is beautiful and strong," becomes "I like myself because I am beautiful and strong."

You are nature. This revised sentence "tricks" your language and reason senses to become consciousness of your inner nature. Can you validate that the changed sentence describes some aspect of yourself? How do you feel about yourself in this light? Does it feel right?

If reading the sentence makes you feel uncomfortable, search your life for one incident or example where it feels right or accurate. If necessary, ask a friend to help you find this part of yourself. Your sentence may be a metaphor. Try to find examples of parts of yourself that accurately match this metaphor. Remember that sometimes you have been taught to deny them. Many people have trouble admitting they are beautiful or strong. Additional activities in these chapters will help you reconnect these parts of you with nature and let nature nurture them so that they feel comfortable. This makes you more immune to nature desensitized people, and they more respectful of you.

When you are with other people, you can do this activity with their inner nature. Find some natural part of yourself that you like or love and see if you can discover and speak to that part of you in another person.

Write down the three most important things you learned from this chapter and.

Write down what, if any, good sensations and feelings were brought on by doing this activity. Can you describe them?

How would you feel about having your ability to sense them taken away?

What effect does this activity have on your sense of self-worth?

Part Three:
Elements of Applied
Ecopsychology

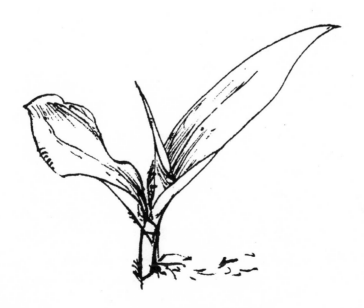

Chapter Ten

Educating and Counseling with Nature:
The Greening of Psychotherapy

*Our multisensory wholeness is the natural foundation
that supports our individuality*

Many outdoor educators and therapists confirm my observation that a reduction of social and psychological problems occurs when our clients/students are in natural areas. We observe that their positive feelings for the environment intensify as well. Perhaps you momentarily experienced this phenomenon when you have had a good experience in nature. This phenomenon parallels the relative absence of psychological problems and insanity found in nature-centered tribal communities and the healthy state of their environment. It suggests that the purpose of modern education, psychology, and psychotherapy is to heal the sensory wounds inflicted by Western civilization's excessive disconnection from the integrity of the global life community. When I teach my participants to use nature-reconnecting activities and ecological reasoning they become more responsible. Their problems wane while their wellness, spirit, and ability to learn increases.

Can sanity truly be defined by Western civilization? Do we promote true sanity if we teach people to support and depend upon irresponsible aspects of our questionable society? As natural beings we are born with the ability to learn nature's wisdom and sanity from nature. What I do is develop activities that let Earth nurture that ability. That is how anybody can help others learn it.

The natural world produces no garbage. On a macro level, it values everything from proton to planet. Nothing in nature is discarded or unwanted, a way of relating that defines unconditional love in action. Scientifically validating and connecting with nature's "unconditional love" and its effects allows us to enjoy it and its benefits.

Since the Spring of 1993, I and my associates have completed an informal study of over 4100 people, mostly aged 16-51, of differing occupations. Our object is to determine if we may observe the effects of separating people from nature by assigning inappropriate words and labels to a person's sensory inner nature. We accomplish this by first asking the study participants:

"When did you first learn to know the color green?"

You might ask yourself that question now. See if your experience parallels our findings.

Our participants responses fall into two main categories:

1. Most participants said they first learned to know the color green when they learned the word green, thereby knowing green by its name or label. For example: "I remember that my parents told me that the name for the color of the grass and trees was green," or "My teacher and labels on the crayons told me they were green."

2. Some participants recognized that they naturally knew and registered green (greenness) as a sense or sensation at birth or before. That kind of knowing is the same natural sensitivity to color found in some insects, plants and microorganisms. For example, one participant said: "Like many other species, I was biologically born knowing green. It is a God thing. As an infant lying on our lawn, I remember naturally distinguishing the green grass from the blue sky and white clouds even though at the time, I couldn't have known the names of their colors." Many studies in developmental psychology show that infants can distinguish colors within the first few months of life. Even though they do not know the names for them, they still know them.

So we know green in two ways:

-by our biological, inborn natural color sense (sensitivity) to green (greenness) that we share with plants and animals that are color sensitive

-by the word-symbol green, a story that labels our sensitivity to green.

However, the study found many examples that confused the question. For example: When Carol was an infant learning to talk, her father, an experimental psychologist, used her as an experiment. He purposely taught her that the name for the color green was orange and the name for orange was green. In time, the words and the colors strongly bonded. Today she is 36 years old and she still gets confused when naming these colors. She still tends to call orange, "green" and green, "orange". Carol can often think about and figure out the correct terms for these colors, but does not automatically know them. Sometimes she feels stupid and stressed for having to think about it and sometimes still mistakes one for the other verbally.

We found several participants who had similar experiences with color, and with other aspects of their biology, too. For example left-handedness:

"The teacher broke my left had by hitting it with a ruler because I wrote with it."

"Unfortunately, as a lefty, I did not learn to write left handed–I learned to write right handed, if you want to call it learning. Today, the only way I can communicate in writing without an interpreter is via typewritten characters."

"Writing with my right hand stressed and depressed me, it resulted in me biting my fingernails and having poor posture."

In light of these findings, we considered the following scenario. It encapsulates what happens to our ability to register greenness.

A teacher tells her first grade class: "Today we are going to learn green," and a child says, "I'll take the day off. I don't need to learn that again, I've naturally known green since before I was born." The teacher responds "Can you read 'green'? Can you write 'green'? Can you spell it or tell me how many times it appears on this chart? If you can't, you are ignorant and illiterate. You will not graduate school, you will not get a good job, you will not be happy. What will your parents do when they learn that you left school today?"

We found that to a greater or lesser degree, our study participants experienced this scenario in their lives. The part of their mentality that naturally knows things through natural senses had learned to experience itself as garbage due to lack of support. How could this vital natural part of them find its identity and self-esteem? In the scenario, the child's inner nature senses abandonment by the people that support the child's life. A child's natural self inherently knows abandonment to be death, for nothing survives without support in nature. In our society, any child's natural security, self-esteem, and self-confidence are at risk until he or she achieves scholastic and occupational skills.

In this scenario, a child would not gain self-worth based on his or her natural skills and intelligence. The child would have to depend upon other aspects of himself or herself to gain self-esteem, support, and confidence.

Our interviews, and our own childhood experiences, disclosed that it was not uncommon for other parts of a child's inherent nature to be dysfunctional through this period since many other parts of a child's inner nature are under assault, too. In many young people we see violence, withdrawal, or dependencies used to relieve the stress we create by not learning to validate nature within and about us. Too often we call this process normal adolescence or rebellion against authority. Too often we carry these kinds of feelings around with us as adults. We are never quite certain what situation might trigger these feelings, so we don't risk participating in many situations that would benefit us and the global life community. That is a way to define irresponsibility and apathy.

Can we learn to feel good about ourselves as natural beings in a nature-separated society? To answer this question we asked each of our study participants to call upon their inner nature, in this case their natural, nonverbal sense of color, to express itself. The vehicle we used for this purpose is the list of color names found on the back cover. The words naming the colors were written in different colored inks (for example, the word "blue" was written in red ink). Participants were asked to quickly go down the color chart list and say aloud the ink colors, not the color names as words. For example, the first color is purple, not red (look at the back cover now if you wish to participate further in this activity).

As a control for this task, we first asked participants to quickly identify blocks of identical ink colors that we painted on a separate page. Only participants that could identify the ink colors were included in the study.

When using the color chart, no participant had difficulty labeling the control blocks of ink colors. However, most participants had difficulty quickly identifying the same ink colors when they spelled out words. The overwhelming tendency was for participant's culturally trained sense of language to dominate and read the color word rather than the actual ink color. It is a graphic demonstration of our language habit or "word addiction." Don't you find that happens for you, too, when you read the chart? In addition, when doing this activity quickly, over 40% of the participants "deluded" themselves in that they spoke a written color name aloud but actually believed they had said the ink color! For example, in the fifth item in the list, Paul believed he read the ink color correctly even though he said the word "blue" while seeing the ink color red. If another person had had not been with him and caught the the error, Paul would not have known that he made it. It's similar to you, the reader, perhaps not noticing that the words "the" and "had" were doubled in the previous sentence until I now alert you to this fact. The difference is that Paul lost awareness of a vital sensory signal from his inner nature, not simply a typographical error. We have identified over 50 distinct sensory signals. They are natural senses. Each is like the sensitivity to greenness that we inherit from nature. They are part of our inner nature.

Our study participants concluded in general:

"My trained habitual dependency on using words overwhelmed my natural senses, an important part of myself. I had trouble expressing my natural ability to recognize color in a non-language way, yet I love color."

One participant offered:

"I love nature yet I have a hard time loving myself. This helps explain why. I am disconnected from nature in me"

Participants never experienced difficulty, tension, conflict, or stress on the last word on the color chart, which is the word green written in green ink. In all cases, "green" written in green ink felt more sensible, relaxing, and attractive than did the other color words. "It feels like a refreshing oasis," said one participant, summing it up. Is that your experience seeing "green" in green, too? Can you validate your experience in your own words? Can you express that "green" written in green ink tends to feel less conflicting, more sensible, relaxing, or comfortable than do the other color words on the chart? With nature's help, you can increase your ability to sense and express this phenomenon.

Our informal study's findings suggest that our awareness, our natural sense of consciousness, is overwhelmingly dominated by words. We are born illiterate, but learn to think primarily through words. Nature-disconnected words separate us from nature within and about us even when we don't want them to, even when we intentionally try not to let this happen. William Irwin Thompson and others have observed that our stories prevent us from seeing things the way they really are, a form of cultural trance or collective hypnosis. To overcome this phenomenon, we must discover ways to use all of our senses to get past our dominating words and stories. In that way, we may find and validate our true colors. Whenever we live out our "greenness" in the distortion of labeling it "orange," we live with undue stress and its destructive personal and social effects. We consist of many "green in orange" capsules of experience that explode and hurt. Whenever we irritate them, they let us feel their stress.

Old Brain and New Brain Thinking

Our study suggests that from early in our lives, nature-separated education conditions us. We are excessively trained to bring the sensory world into our awareness by labeling it with language abstractions, words, symbols, and image stories. In addition, we learn to validate the reasonable meanings of these abstractions in our culture. I say "excessively" because the study shows that our language stories throw us out of balance and stress us (green in orange). They overpower our inner nature, sometimes to the point of deluding us (like Paul saying blue and thinking he said red). They challenge us to discover how to reduce conflict in our personal lives (green in green). At every moment of our waking lives, we psychologically live in one of these 3 states of being: uncomfortably stressed, deluded into denial, or happily unconflicted.

Neurological researchers find that two different natural sense groups in two different parts of the brain are at work when we "know" something natural like the color green. Because of the evolutionary history of these parts of the brain, one part is called the old brain. The other is called the new brain, or neocortex.

The Old Brain

Our natural sense of color enables our screen of consciousness to experience color as "greenness," an unlabeled, nonverbal sensation or feeling. The natural sense of color, along with at least 50 other natural sensory clusters, lie in the large, anciently evolved "old-brain". The old-brain registers non-language tensions, sensations, feelings, and emotions. It makes up approximately 87% of the total brain and is the home of many different sense groups that are also found throughout the natural world. These are the senses listed in chapter five.

Researchers show that most of our old brain sensitivities we inherit from, and share with, the plant, animal and even mineral kingdoms. These natural senses are facts as real as rocks, oceans, and gravity. For example, our desire to breathe is an attraction to air that is as real as the air; our hunger for food is an attraction as real as an apple. In nature, a multisensory concert of natural sensitivities synergize to create the balanced "natural sense" that is nature's beauty, peace, and wisdom. It is important to recognize that the conflict of green in orange is absent in nature because nature does not use a verbal, literate language or story that abstracts reality. Rather, nature practices reality. We seldom learn to honor that nature is a beautiful, intelligent illiteracy.

The New Brain

Two senses, language and reason, lie in our small, more recently evolved, "new-brain" (neocortex). These two senses give our screen of consciousness the ability to know our old brain sensory experiences (like registering color) as a culturally correct word, label, or story, such as the word "green" or "orange." We train the new brain to make it feel reasonable for us to know colors as a words, to know sensations as abstractions with the correct name.

The new-brain makes up only about 13% of the total brain and does not reach biological maturity until late adolescence. It creates, experiences, validates, and processes culturally trained symbolism: language, letters, words, numbers, drawings, logic, abstractions, and stories. They often play like a movie on our inner screen of consciousness. We have the ability to change the movie. We call this ability "thinking." Society teaches us to mostly think and reason in nature-disconnected new brain symbols and stories. With respect to nature, we are often unaware of our thinking's connectedness or disconnectedness.

Our new brain stories presently manage the natural world within us and around us. Are we satisfied with their effects? Can we teach the new brain to do better?

Trusting This Study

Some people don't trust the findings of the scientific world, they are never sure of their accuracy. In this study, you need not depend upon science to discover facts. You can find your own truth. Look at the color chart again. Can you distinguish a difference in your comfort or stress level between seeing green in green and seeing the rest of the colors written in different colored inks? Can you trust what you sense, your experience, your feelings in the immediate moment? If not, what can you trust?

This study suggests that from early in our lives, the ancient sense of color, lying in the old-brain, enables us to naturally register the color green as a pure sensation. Our sense of color experiences green directly as a natural, non-languaged, unadulterated, unedited, unmediated feeling. The old brain brings to sensory awareness how we naturally feel. It is often called our inner nature, our inner self. Sometimes this sensory wisdom is misnamed our "inner child," even though it is an essence of Earth itself. When we operate from our old brain's natural sensations and feelings, Western culture often devalues us by saying that we are being too emotional, sensitive, childlike, or intuitive. However, natural senses and feelings are of, by, and from nature. Their role can best be measured, without prejudice, by their long term survival effects. Remember, these include their known ability to create an optimum of life, diversity, and beauty without producing runaway garbage, insanity, or war.

In the smaller new-brain, the neocortex, Western culture often trains the senses of language and reason to apply cultural words, labels, or stories to the natural senses. We teach the new brain that it is reasonable to know greenness as the written or spoken word green, or verde (Spanish), or vert (French), or other words in different languages and cultures. We applaud our intelligence, our new brain, for doing so. When we operate from senses of language and reason, we often say proudly that we are literate, cerebral, sensible, abstract, cognitive, reasonable, logical, intelligent, educated, or thoughtful. In applied ecopsychology, we create an additional story. It says it is also intelligent to reconnect our old brain with nature and learn and speak from that experience.

The depressing anger, anxiety, and sadness produced by our new brain mislabeling, overlooking, or rejecting our old brain's natural senses and feelings stress us. That stress fuels our problems at many levels. We are not islands. As we remain consciously estranged from the wisdom, spirit, and unconditional love of the natural world, our negative personal, social, and environmental indicators rise. Even outdoor education does not resolve these problems when it does not teach us how to consciously have our new brain validate and fulfill our inner nature's need to be connected, loved, and nurtured by nature.

To reverse our troubles, we must learn to reconnect with nature. We must learn to effectively communicate with nature in order to know its ways. To accomplish this, we must either figure out how to teach the natural world to speak English or we must learn to understand its multiple-sensory nonverbal language. The latter course makes the most sense since we already know nature's sensory callings. We inherit them. They are part of our old brain. Consider the following example:

> I have never met Hank, yet I feel very close to him. He used to write professionally. Five years ago, he was in an auto accident and suffered whiplash. Despite six operations and chemical and psychotherapy, he has been in pain continuously since the accident. That stopped his writing career. Six weeks ago he began doing the nature connecting activities as part of our e-mail nature reconnecting course. While doing the activities, Hank felt relief from headache pain for the first time in five years. He was so excited, so thankful, that he wrote me and said he wanted to write about this wonderful experience. In his excitement, his thoughts ran to how he might write about

what was happening to him as he did the course activities. What magazine or editor might be interested in hearing about it? What were the deadline dates for article submissions? Suddenly, his headaches reappeared. He had let his new brain stressfully invade rather than support his old brain connections with nature. Sadly, Hank wrote me that he might never be able to write again. I pointed out that he had been writing successfully on the course for six weeks in ways that diminished his pain. Why not just continue that kind of writing since it worked? If necessary, he could find somebody to take care of the submissions. Hank agreed and completed the course. He then taught it to others, produced some wonderful essays, and has since fulfilled professional writing assignments.

Once again, think about what our world would be like if 600 million people had RWN experiences daily; experiences that were similar to Hank's involving nature and the community. That thought is the essence of the RWN factor and that thought is not ours alone. In some form, the sense in that thought is shared by every member of global life community, no matter their cultural differences or species. It is the love of life, an essence of being Hank.

Activity 10: Natural Old-Brain Connecting

Discover and strengthen your non-languaged sensory inner nature. Go a natural area. Ask for its permission for you to become involved with it. Gain its consent to help you with this activity.

Without using language, try to connect your non-verbal, sensory inner nature with the non-languaged natural world. Seek the nurturing "mother" community where your natural sensory faculties originated, evolved, and feel at home. Reconnect your old brain to nature by simply sensing natural attractions in this natural area (colors, moods, loves, textures, motions, forms, variations, touch, taste, smells, sounds, atmospheres, contrasts, etc.) without assigning words or ideas to them. This is nonverbal connecting, similar to how the natural world knows itself. It is a challenge. If your new brain wrangles your consciousness to habitually or addictively drift to thoughts, stories, or to labeling the natural area, tie it up from doing so by repeating the word "non-language" or "nameless" over and over again as you sense the area. Note whether or not that makes a difference. Experiment, try to find a word that works best for you. Sometimes it is helpful just to forcefully tell your sense of language to be quiet. These procedures allow your non-language awareness to exist in the moment. You sense more completely in that moment. Thank your non-languaged old brain for that faculty. Moving through the area without concentrating on any one thing also helps you make nonverbal contact.

Some participant's reactions:

"I felt detached and free, almost like I was walking in a dream."

"Everything became more intense, I felt more connected."

"Suddenly I could hear sounds that had been there all along, but which I had ignored."

"It felt like jumping in a lake, I felt my surroundings, I floated in them."

Write down the three most important things you learned from this activity. Write down what, if any, good sensations and feelings were brought on by doing this activity. Can you describe them? How would you feel about having your ability to sense them taken away? What effect does this activity have on your sense of self-worth?

Chapter Eleven

The Green/Orange to Green/Green Formula

*Without experiencing them by name, we don't believe
our 53 natural senses are real.*

To manage stress in balanced ways, we must learn to counteract the adverse effects of our new-brain, nature-separated stories. We must learn to experience and appreciate the beneficial nature- connective properties of the old brain.

At any time, we can choose to do activities in natural areas that allow the differences between the old and new brain to sensibly find common ground. The activities let nature's on-site intelligence help reduce our runaway inner stress, conflict, and wanting. These stresses produce our greed and insensitive abusiveness of people and the environment.

What to Do: Reconnecting with nature psychologically recognizes that nature beautifully sustains life through nonverbal attachment relationships. They consist of sensory attraction bonds that organize and build themselves without using our new brain stories. This psychology is simple and fun because it lets tangible contact with nature's intelligence do most of the work. To participate, we thoughtfully say (new brain) what we feel in nature (old brain). The process consists of four elements:

1. VALIDATE SENSORY KNOWLEDGE: We validate that our inborn ability to sense and feel is of, by, and from the old brain and nature; that sensation and feeling attractions, like color or thirst, are facts that in nature are nameless but as real as Earth itself.

2. NATURE CONNECT: In parks, backyards, or even with potted plants, we thankfully gain permission from an attractive natural area to visit it and do harmless activities that produce tangible sensory contacts with nature, including nature within others.

3. VALIDATE NATURAL FEELINGS: When we feel comfortable in a connection with nature we validate that we sense a green in green (G/G) attraction connection blending the new and old brain. We validate this connection by translating our experience into words that reasonably convey our experience. We read these words to ourselves and share them with other people. This thoughtfully engages our new brain in acknowledging the reasonableness and relationship building value of our old brain connection with nature. Our good feelings are nature's way of telling us that we are in contact with NIAL and our new brain's story is supporting our old brain's connections with nature.

When we feel uncomfortable in a connection with nature, we validate that, as on the color chart, we are like green in orange (G/O). A conflict exists between the new and old brain. Our stressful feelings are nature's way of telling us that our new brain's stories are not supporting our old brain's connections to nature.

4. BRING G/G'S VALUE INTO CONSCIOUSNESS: We help our new brain develop reasonable respect for our new feelings by asking ourselves if we are willing to give up having these good feelings. We ask if it makes sense to have them removed from our lives and if not, why not?

In activity 6, stressful feelings result from implementing the "stop breathing" story that disconnects us from the plant. Green in green is the feeling from the story that reconnects us with the plant. In the "wrapped hand" activity 8, green in orange is the sensation of the hand disconnected by the sweater wrapped around it. G/G is the sensation enjoyed by the unwrapped "natural" hand.

Nature is alive, attractive, nameless, and always intelligently changing by fulfilling natural attractions. No two moments or things in nature are ever the same. Once the natural attraction is established, it grows through further attraction fulfillments. As this happens, we need to let the new brain validate additional attractive connections. For survival, we and nature constantly need and enjoy connections with all of life and its changes, not just one connection in a single moment.

Each time we connect with nature, we not only establish new relationships with people and Earth, we also extend our new brain's ability to establish, trust, and seek them. In this process, our new brain applauds our old brain's natural gift for manifesting comforting feelings in nature. It also applauds itself for being reasonable enough to orchestrate comfortable reconnecting moments. With this nurturing and support, our natural senses increasingly awaken and provide the new brain with nature's additional support and wisdom. In time, the process becomes a habit, an enjoyable, multisensory nature-connected way of thinking. It beneficially produces responsible stories and relationships, personally and globally. Anytime you go to a natural area, you can feel better and reinforce the process. You may do this with people's inner nature, too, as is exemplified by sharing with others what happens in an activity.

An important aspect of the green/orange to green/green transition is that it begins with consciously seeking our natural attractions to nature by obtaining permission to visit from the natural area. This is vital. It grounds the activities in sensitivity, good feelings, and language emanating from natural attractions. These feelings motivate, support, and energize the new brain to safely participate. They provide support from nature. It overcomes the resistance and fear attached to creating a nature-connected way of thinking and relating that often goes against the ingrained "conquer nature" story of the civilizing process.

Bathed and supported by pleasurable non-language attractions, the activities safely carry participants through the stories that block the process. A real-life example of the process is detailed in the appendix.

The Wranglers

One big contribution that the nature reconnecting process makes is that it automatically brings into our consciousness the past or present situations that prevent us from feeling green in green (Superego, Parent, Authority etc.) The stories and people in these situations act as wranglers. They treat us like cattle. They do not ask our permission to honor their demands nor request that we thoughtfully consider them. This especially happens when we are children. These wrangling situations, or the feelings activated by our memories of them, "round us up, herd and drive us" into the wrangler's stories, attitudes, and relationships. When dissatisfied with our plight, we have difficulty changing it because we were not involved in building it. We still depend upon or fear the wrangler. We are unaware of the experiences, fears, reasoning, and process used by wranglers to construct or modify the stories that direct us. We were wrangled, not invited or educated, into them. They did not ask or gain our permission to enter our psyche. They are stories imposed by parents, teachers, ministers, friends, institutions, advertising, and the many other authorities that prod our lives. Within and around us, wranglers supplant our sense of reason.

When we are consciously sustaining relationships through an uncomfortable story, a wrangler within us is stressfully wrangling us into a G/O feeling. For example, the people who teach us industrial society's "conquer nature" survival stories are wranglers. As long as our relationship with them remains intact within our psyche, they wrangle us into living our excessively nature separated lives.

It is important to recognize that what we call habitual or conditioned thoughts and feelings are misnomers. They are actually moments in our lives when hidden wranglers within our psyche goad us into certain ways of thinking and relating. Reconnecting with nature methods and materials let nature itself touch these internal wranglers and educate them. The process enables wranglers within us to feel, acknowledge, and welcome natural attractions. It is as if we take our wranglers and do the first few activities with them.

When doing the reconnecting with nature activities, we must prevent ourselves from wrangling nature in ourselves, natural areas or other people. We accomplish this by asking nature's permission to become involved with nature. We seek nature's consent to help us with the activity before proceeding. Natural senses then make their own sense. They come into play and signal us to either continue because it feels safe, attractive, and responsible, or to do the activity in some other attractive area. In the process, our inner nature learns to demand the same respect from new brain stories and wranglers.

Often our memories of wranglers and their stories are uncomfortable and therein lies the remarkable strength of the G/O to G/G process. Because the process starts with supportive connection experiences in natural areas and people, it feeds and energizes itself from our wrangled G/O discomforts while reducing them. It thrives by letting nature itself change green in orange discomfort into green in green comfort. This is exactly how nature flourishes. Nature feeds on, and recycles, "waste" products. Nature transforms our wastes into food, water, air, and beauty that sustain it and us. It also does this with our psychologically unhealthy and mind-polluting conflicts.

Reconnecting with nature activities ask nature to recycle our discontents. They ecopsychologically take us from outrage to action. We gain the wisdom, energy and support from natural areas that motivates us to address each G/O situation we encounter. We participate. All this is a gift from nature as free as fresh air and sunshine. Just as we can reasonably discover the "sanity" of green-in-green on a color chart diagram, we can find it in reality by seeking positive relationships in nature, including people's sensory inner nature. The process identifies our wranglers and reeducates them. As we participate, wranglers dissipate.

The cognitive aspect of reconnecting with nature consists of the new brain learning to trust and validate the use of nature connecting activities as well as understanding and validating how the green in orange to green-in-green transition works. It learns why the process is trustable and how it changes the G/O stories that block us from enjoying G/G. Reconnecting with nature recognizes that in our society our wrangled childhood conditions us to be conscious through new brain stories, not through sensory old brain nature connections. Personal and global wellness depend upon which stories we choose or create moment by moment.

The essence of reconnecting with nature is that its activities always enable the new brain to include tangible, nonverbal, old brain sensory connections with nature in people and places. They become part of every story or relationship. In our increasingly nature disconnected world, nothing short of this makes sense. It is nonsense to expect to use a disconnected process and not be disconnected sooner or later. It makes sense to recognize that whenever we receive gratification from doing something that does not involve tangible contact with nature, subconsciously we learn, that we don't need nature for our lives. In this sense, even our comfortable moments watching videos that promote nature secretly tell us that we can continue to enjoy life without directly connecting with nature. Who amongst us feels that they emotionally need nature when they are already fulfilled by nature videos? Remaining disconnected from true nature keeps us in the emotional rut we've been in for centuries. Every time we travel that rut, we deepen it.

Sentiently reconnecting with genuine nature, is an ecopsychological ladder that takes us out of our rut. Each rung of the ladder is a responsible participatory relationship with nature that takes us one step closer to long term wellness. It creates global wellness by creating immediate wellness moment by moment. The ladder makes rational connections with Earth that are far more genuine than the many stories and fantasies that wrangle us down civilization's wayward path.

The color chart study is not only an experience, it is also a metaphor for how and why reconnecting with nature works anywhere. The study shows that in Western civilization we already have the know-how we need to get out of our rut. It shows that our cultural stories already contain the following common knowledge:

At birth we are biologically at one with nature. We are born illiterate because nature is a nonverbal way of knowing and being .

Early in life, society applauds, educates, and wrangles our new brain to be literate, to learn and think in language. We become bonded to being conscious of the world through written and spoken stories. However, our old brain and the natural environment remain a non-language relationship; a self sustaining, interconnected, sensory way of intelligently knowing and being that organizes, promotes, and regenerates itself.

As we mature, in any given moment of our lives our stories have the capacity to bring to our screen of consciousness acculturated new brain stories or old brain natural sensations .

We live, learn, and bond to living indoors, to creating enjoyment while separated from nature. We learn to applaud stories about how to manage the world so that we may continue to enjoy living our nature separated lives. Society conditions us to know who we are personally and collectively from our stories and their nature conquering beliefs, settings, and ways. To sustain our artificial indoor world, our stories wrangle us to assault and conquer our sensory nature connected old brain ways of knowing and thinking along with the natural environment. We cannot do one without doing the other for both are nature. When we call our natural senses and feelings anything other than "nameless nature," we open the door for misleading stories.

Our new brain stories always have the capacity to transition from dissociative G/O stories to connective G/G stories. We can discern one from the other because G/O stories lead us to conflict and feeling uncomfortable. G/G stories lead us to the comfortable feelings of harmony with nature in people and places. We come to our senses personally and globally by letting the stress we feel move us to reconnect with nature and enjoy the attractive comfort we feel from green-in-green.

We are aware that we may find comfort where nature has created it, in the natural environment and in people's unadulterated inner nature. We enjoy the rewards of our transition by making tangible contact with nature within and around us. We know we are often mislead by wrangler's stories parading before us. For example, advertisements that show people enjoying cigarettes while sitting in the grandeur of a natural area. We may think we are connecting with nature by watching pictures of nature instead of enjoying genuine contact with a natural area. We are often unaware that pictures of nature do not contain nor convey the multisensory wisdom we may obtain from a natural area.

We know that for the survival of life and ourselves, we must participate in and support our beneficial interdependent relationship with Earth.

Reconnecting with nature is a green in green story that we may choose to enact by participating in nature reconnecting activities. Each activity takes us from G/O to G/G and since we own the activity, we can use it anywhere, time and time again to the same effect. In addition, we can teach the activity to others.

The reconnecting with nature story gives our new brain good reasons to do these activities. It explains to the new brain that we deserve to have good feelings because we are alive. Our good feelings result from our natural attraction senses being fulfilled as they sustain life. That's how nature works. The new brain chooses to feel good and make sense of our natural sensory relationships because it obtains permission and makes it reasonable and safe to do so. It feels right and it produces responsible short and long term effects. The new brain learns that by choosing to reconnect with nature we can choose to feel good without being abused by wranglers or becoming abusive wranglers. Nature is safe and supportive. It does not communicate in stories that can mislead us.

Reconnecting with nature is effective because when we actually reconnect with the non-language world of nature, our mind automatically brings to consciousness experiences and feelings from our past that wrangle us from being connected to nature. These experiences are no longer hidden from us in our subconscious. This phenomenon has been documented by Dr. Wilder Penfield in open brain surgery where the new brain in an awake anesthetized patient has been physically stimulated with a probe and a specific story/memory with attached feelings registers in consciousness. Until it is over, the memory feels so real in consciousness that it feels like it's happening in the present. The feelings cannot be recognized by the patient as part of a story/memory from the past. In the non-language world of nature, these feelings/sensations afford protection by bringing to our screen of consciousness past experiences that recognized and dealt with a similar threatening situation. The nature-reconnecting process supportively brings these experiences on to our screen of consciousness for our new brain's consideration. Then we learn from them and our many natural senses intelligently deal with them.

The beauty of reconnecting is that the process is built on supportive green-in-green feelings and Earth's natural intelligence. When we engage in activities to relieve stress of any kind, our inner nature sensitivity to natural attractions innately selects the places and situations in nature that it needs for healing. Our inner nature identifies and reconnects to them for it is them and it longs for them. For example, when we stop drinking and disconnect from water, the sense of thirst begins to tell us that we need water, not dust or air. Water becomes attractive; it tastes better, too. During any given moment that we connect to nature, certain natural things always appear to beckon and feel attractive while others don't. We learn to reinforce their ability to do this by acknowledging this gift.

In nature, the immediate moment's attractiveness, or lack of it, is significant. It always contains a special wisdom to support our personal growth and relationships. In this way, nature reconnecting activities are similar to using a psychological test as a therapeutic experience and education.

Color Chart Examples

Based on participation in the color chart study, the following are some examples of people in various intensities and stages of participation in the G/O to G/G nature-reconnecting process. I have changed the names of the individuals they describe:

In real life, when Linette feels stressed she goes to the park. Alone or with friends, she gains its permission to use nature reconnecting activities to replace her stress with good feelings. The process enables her to obtain support from nature in herself, the environment, and her friends. It gives her insights as to why she was stressed as well as a vehicle to improve her stressful relationships. When Linette views the color chart, she chooses to stay on the green in green line much of the time. She recognizes that it is more comfortable and sensible than the green in orange lines. Occasionally she chooses G/O for the fun and challenge of it, with the knowledge that she can always safely return to G/G. She feels thankful for the ability to feel G/G and says it feels like an oasis.

While doing the color chart, Paul recognizes that he feels stress because he lets the activity wrangle him. He intends to say the ink color red but he rushes and instead says the written word "blue" However, Paul has learned to give his inner nature the time and space to say the ink color red and be sure that he has said it, rather than be subject to his tendency to read the word blue. Paul has learned to sensibly, painstakingly fulfill his intentions here and elsewhere, and not be wrangled by stressful stories that lead to undesirable effects.

Sarah is similar to Paul but she often tries to relieve her disconnected feelings by pointing out to others how and when they are green in orange. She invasively puts her relationships at risk by being a wrangler. She becomes an authoritative teacher or parent substitute bearing discomforting news or telling people what to do without first getting their consent.

Art did not trust the color chart and how he reacted to it until he found experts that validated what he experienced with it. He needed some authority with credentials to tell him it was all right for him to trust the difference in feelings he experienced between G/O and G/G on the chart.

Carol was wrangled to learn the color orange as the word green and vice versa when she first learned to talk. She is bonded to this way of knowing and until it becomes a discomforting concern that she tries to correct, she will repeat this habitual error again and again. To change this error, she may choose to learn to do what Paul and Linette do with their stress, to use nature itself to relive her orange in green experiences, disregard the wrangler, and gain support to select and enjoy green-in-green from nature.

Bill's pain from his abusive disconnected past relationships now color most of his potentially positive experiences and makes them into stressful stories. He relates to others abusively, as if the immediate moment was harsh and causing him pain. Bill chooses orange in green ways of relating in order to explain to himself why he feels pain. He chemically abuses himself to tranquilize the discomfort of his wrangling immediate and past relationships. He considers therapy as nonsense because he does not acknowledge any personal problems, only that others pick on him. By court order, Bill is being treated with medications and various therapies while in and out of jail.

The G/O to G/G process is summed up in Al. He said that he never learned the color gray because when his parents originally showed him the color gray, he said it was black. They told him he was wrong in a harsh way that wrangled him, and then showed him a lighter gray, which he said was white. He was again told he was wrong. He never felt comfortable identifying gray for it carried with it the risk of feeling wrong. Today, at the age of 53 years, Al still does not know the color gray. He still calls gray either black or white. At a nature-connecting workshop, when Al went to a natural area to find immediate attractions. On each of 5 different occasions, the natural things that unconsciously attracted him were colored gray: rocks, bark, lichens, sticks, and driftwood. His inner nature seemed to automatically be using moments in nature to bring up and resolve an ancient conflict with his parents that disconnected him from gray in gray. As he continued doing the activities, he gained enough support from the environment and the workshop group to risk calling he objects gray. His reward was an easing of his stress about his situation and enjoying the spontaneous approval he received from his new brain and the workshop participants. He was sure that with practice he could feel comfortable identifying the color gray, but he did not think he would spend time doing it. It was not as high a priority as were the challenges of his daily life as a mental health worker and environmental consultant. He did say however, that very high priority situations did exist that needed immediate relief. He noted that over 80% of the population suffers from stress and almost 90% feels discontent about how we treat the environment. He felt that reconnecting with nature would work wonders in solving these aggravating personal and environmental problems and that's where he would put his energies.

The color chart activity pinpoints a significant challenge we face if we are to reverse our disorders. Our old brain, when not directly reconnected to nature, is overridden by new brain stories and often is unaware of it. For example, we tend to say the written word on the chart before saying the ink color. We often say the word and think we've said the color, especially when we are stressed or tired. This misleads those of us who seek guidance and strength from our inner being. We must be sure time and energy are available to affirm that we make conscious contact with our 53 non-languaged old brain senses (the ink colors), and not false words wranglers have attached to them. Following culturally polluted guidance is a disease, not a remedy.

The advantage of the G/O to G/G experience is that it is built on non-language relationships with nature. This assures that adverse new brain stories will not contaminate the relationship. It gives a natural purity to the spirit or higher power we seek. It enables us to authentically touch our natural origins, community, and creation. St. Basil attempted to convey this when he said: "Wherever you may go, the least plant may bring you clear remembrance of the Creator." However, his new brain story influenced what he said. There is no such thing in nature as a "least" plant. In nature, everything has its own as well as a common integrity; that eliminates garbage. No one thing is greater or lesser than another. That is just another one of our stories, not nature's way.

The world and its people are at risk as a result of our stories that excessively separate us from nature's truths. Reconnecting with nature addresses this problem. It is a simple hands-on system that teaches the new brain that it makes sense to make time and space for the old brain to safely reconnect with nature, and thoughtfully validate the stories arising from the process. These stories let you think for yourself because they contain nature's sensory intelligence and support. Appendix A offers valuable guidelines and examples of how to achieve this. The G/O to G/G process described there promotes mental and environmental health for the two are identical, as the following example illustrates:

In 1936, Charlie, a left-handed 6-year old child, enters the public school system and is wrangled to write with his right hand. From the tension of this requirement, Charlie begins to bite his nails until they bleed. Five years later, while in sixth grade, Charlie is allowed to write with his left hand, but his nail biting habit continues for 57 years. He is living under the influence of a hidden wrangler that is alive and well within him. In 1993, at the age of 63, Charlie enters a program where he learns and practices nature-connecting activities. They encourage his inner nature, including his left-handedness, to validate itself by connecting to real nature, to attractive natural areas and objects. Many months later, someone asks Charlie why he bites his nails and Charlie explains his history to them. A week later Charlie notices that, with no effort on his part, his nails have started to grow. Without realizing it, he had re-educated his inner wrangler and broken a 57 year habit that has never returned. In the process, he further bonded with the natural environment.

Again think about what our world would be like if 600 million people in it had daily RWN experiences with nature and their community, experiences that were similar to those Charlie had. That thought is the essence of the RWN factor and it is shared by every member of the global life community, no matter what their cultural differences or species. The sense in that thought is the love of life, a green-in-green essence of Charlie and of life.

Activity 11: New Brain Connecting

Go to an attractive natural area. Ask for its permission to become involved with it, gain its consent to help you with this activity.

If the area remains attractive, repeat the activity to know this natural area non-verbally. Then, new-brain connect to each part of it of which you become aware. Do this by reasonably labeling that you are consciously connecting to, not just labeling the objects themselves. Focus your new brain on the whole of the moment including yourself. Accomplish this by calling each thing you sense "a connection experience." For example, if you see a leaf, call the leaf a connection. If a bird's color, motion, distance, beauty, or song catches your attention, also call it a connection. Each sensory contact is a connection.

All conscious contact is a form of natural connection. It reasonably brings the natural sensory connection process into new-brain language awareness. This enables the new-brain to consciously make sense, register, and validate the existence of many natural sensory connections as well as how they contribute to our welfare. Some participant's reactions:

"Saying 'connection' helped me blend my new brain with nature. The woods felt more attractive and stronger than usual."

"It backfired, I got into enjoying a non-language way of knowing and the word 'connection' interrupted it."

"Saying the word 'connection' seemed right, it made sense...it did not mislead me."

"Actually, it did not seem to make a difference when I did it, but after the activity it felt right."

Write down the three most important things you learned from this activity. Write down what, if any, good sensations and feelings were brought on by doing this activity. Can you describe them? How would you feel about having your ability to sense them taken away? What effect does this activity have on your sense of self-worth?

Chapter Twelve

Disconnection and the Tropicmakers

The stress created by detaching our natural senses from nature stems from the creation of nature-separated environments.

Nature centered thinking applies the principles of ecopyschology. It includes and honors contact with nature's nameless, intelligent, attraction loves (NIAL). This psychological consciousness is one that we naturally sense and enjoy. Whenever our new brain's words do not accurately describe what we sense and feel while in nature's presence, we live in the stress of some wrangling story that has drifted away from nature's unifying ways and wisdom.

Nature-centered thinking recognizes that nature purposely created and gives us the ability to know and feel the difference between green-in-green and green-in-orange. At any given moment we can choose to reconnect with nature and regain the comfort of being in equilibrium. This lets nature sentiently flow through us and nurture us. It beneficially regulates our relationships with nature in people and places by enlisting the NIAL of the ages that produced them. In addition, it enables us to build responsible relationships with people by sharing G/G with them verbally and in community.

One good way to discover the essence of something is to try to change it. We are born as attached to nature as our arm is attached to our body. Our way of life tries to change our inborn relationship to nature into the indoor tenets of Western civilization. We learn to spend less than one day per lifetime in tune with nature. We vaguely sense the pain of our disconnection like a pilot dropping bombs on people 20,000 feet below. We live in stories desensitized to their hurtful effects.

Like the connecting strands of cheese that appear when you disconnect a slice of pizza from the whole pie, each of our nature-connected senses is stretched, torn, or otherwise injured by excessive separation from nature. The hurt this produces seeks tranquilization and protection from further aggravation. The torn sense needs to be expressed and satisfied in some way. This nature disconnection phenomenon is the source of our runaway social and environmental dilemmas. It helps explain why we can't easily control these problems. Each problem is nature's cohesiveness calling attention to a disconnection. Personal and environmental problems are often either a plea for help or a release or sedative for the lack of natural gratification we feel. To stop the problem behavior is to risk bringing on the pain. To prevent this from happening, we may even deny that a problem exists. This does not occur when using nature-reconnecting activities. They work by reconnecting with NIAL and nature does the rest.

We have disconnected from NIAL to the point that, like a person raised in a cult, most of us don't realize that an intelligent, fun part of us has disappeared from our screen of consciousness. We keep disconnection pain out of our consciousness by avoiding awareness of it. We avoid personal contacts or injure people and the environment in order not to aggravate our pain. We don't allow ourselves to contact or feel our effects. When we do, we sense despair and grief.

When we feel that something is missing from our life, it is often some important fulfillment of NIAL. This is what people mean when they say that our extreme indoor upbringing brainwashes us to its limited ways and perceptions. Brainwashing can be seen as a forcible indoctrination to induce a child to give up natural, inherent attitudes and accept regimented, disconnected ways of thinking.

The belief that we may continue surviving by conquering nature is part of our problem. Like any habit, it will not go away easily. But even if tomorrow that idea disappeared within and around us, our relationships would be difficult to change. We are emotionally, socially, and economically bonded to our indoor relationships. Wranglers detach our natural senses from nature and reattach them to our indoor ways and stories. The senses gain a reduced gratification there. They adjust to compromising themselves, to obtaining immediate satisfactions in nature-estranged ways, regardless of whether these ways may or may not satisfy our sense of reason. To make changes, we need to regain support. We must not only make changes in our story, we must un-bond from our irresponsible patterns and be open to thoughtfully trusting and enjoying our old brain's wise natural attractions to nature. These attachments provide responsible support. They help us become whole and more fulfilled because they are not wrangled by our society's story. Instead they have the freedom to interact with nature's ways. This process is reasonable. It responsibly generates good feelings by satisfying our natural sense of reason.

Too often, we overlook the power of our attachments to our new brain stories. Think about Carol, the woman whose father taught her that the word for greenness was orange, and vice versa. Her experience shows that our perceptions are not simply immediate sensory inputs. The world around us registers on our screen of consciousness as a sensory input plus the story attached to it. Carol senses green yet automatically thinks and says orange. Until the glue between seeing green and the word orange is dissolved and the word green is glued in to replace orange, Carol is conscious of a separate reality than the rest of us.

What we call education does a lot of gluing. We think by considering and rearranging glued stories, not by responsibly un-gluing and regluing them based on sensory experiences that include contact with nature. For this reason, we continue to think our way into repeating the problems we already have. Education has yet to show that it practices the process of un-gluing and regluing when we discover we are on an irresponsible path.

There are 53 different kinds of redirected sensory glue that make our indoor connections. Each is the attraction power of one of the natural senses that has been disconnected from nature and reconnected to some indoor substitute. Indoor counseling often un-glues and then re-bonds us to our nature-disconnected path. It, too, skirts input from nature's intelligence.

Nature-centered psychology shows that to make reasonable changes it is reasonable to use nature reconnecting activities. The activities have the power to let nature un-glue us from irresponsible fulfillments by gratifying NIAL in us. The activities then re-bond us to nature and let nature's multisensory intelligence help resolve our problems. The process enables our rejuvenated natural senses to help our sense of reason understand. This appears to be preposterous in our society's nature-disconnected thinking. It threatens our new brain's training to conquer nature, so we give the process little value or support. However, as Eric Fromm and many others note: just because the same mental pathology is shared by thousands of people, it does not make these people sane. Fortunately, nature sustains its sanity by acting from its 53 sensory intelligences in congress with each other. Nature reconnecting activities allow supportive attraction experiences in nature to register this process in our consciousness and modify our old stories. The sensible gratification we obtain as we transition from G/O to G/G motivates us to continue the process and responsibly support our lives and all of life. That is how and why we generate and deserve to have good feelings.

"Tropicmaking"

Evidence processed by anthropologists and archeologists suggests that originally the natural world supported humanity in the tropical areas. There, moment by moment, our survival dictated that we connect with and learn from nature. Ancient peoples learned to survive through nature's opportunities. They learned to develop reasonable stories that described how nature worked. These stories made them conscious of what natural opportunities presented themselves.

As our reasoning and language senses developed stories that celebrated nature's ways, we became increasingly conscious of our old brain's connections with nature and the sensations and feelings of being connected. Our natural senses imbued human thinking and civilization. The process supplied additional survival knowledge, support, and cooperative life-giving boundaries. Today, responsible societies still support this sensible nature-connected tradition and way of thinking. As a result, they don't promote our runaway problems.

Western civilization's shortsighted nature-conquering story wrangles our sense of consciousness. This story developed when our cultural ancestors encountered situations that challenged their innate tropical-survival way of knowing and being. As climatic conditions changed either through glaciation or by our migrations into new areas, the ancients discovered that by combining their new-brain senses of language, reason, and consciousness, they could conceive and create artificial, tropic-simulating "closets." These consisted of agricultural and indoor environments, free of the natural world's life giving tension and relaxation fluctuations. For example, senses of temperature, sight, and place could be satisfied by building a fire rather than by waiting for the sun to shine, the weather to change, or by moving to a warmer area. Experience by experience, our cultural ancestors became conscious that, through their new brain story, they could survive in any environment they could build tropic-like closets. Through their stories they could also remember the gifts of the tropics such as fruited trees. Technology could make that memory into a reality in the form of a fruit orchard. Humans became artificial Tropicmakers. Their sense of consciousness became conscious of reason, language, and itself as major survival factors. Together, these three senses formed the new brain. It became aware of the story that it could promote human survival by changing the natural environment to fit its tropicmaking thinking. Out of context with nature's ways, new brain reasoning and language could create survival stories that were out of context with nature. These stories may be the only thing in the Universe that is out of context with nature. Enacting these stories gratified some of the ancient's old brain sensory attractions. These natural senses un-bonded from nature and re-bonded to new brain's capacity to create survival stories. That capacity, not nature, became synonymous with survival. The new brain's story making ability observed itself, not nature, to have the wisdom and power of a god. It became the wrangler of the global life community.

Out of ignorance and arrogance, our cultural ancestors created and heeded stories that removed them from immediate moments living and learning in nature. Their new stories applauded their "intelligence and creativity" to create stories that sustained survival independently of nature's whims and wisdom. They were deluded into believing that they no longer needed immediate connections to the intelligence of creation They survived because of the wisdom of new brain stories that played like movies in their heads. They lived in and revered their nature-disconnected stories, spoken stories that were foreign to nature. They physically trespassed on nature's ways and imposed their abuse on the land. No other species understood or consented to these stories. Their stories led them out of nature's paradise. Instead of nature being their source, it became their resource. A story from the scriptures portrays this nature disconnection process as the sin of eating of the tree of knowledge in the Garden of Eden. Some geographers give it a different name. They call it the desertification of the Middle East and Sahara.

In time, our cultural ancestor's prime story became "To survive we must conquer nature and build artificial tropics." Deaf to the self-regulating balanced intelligence of their old brain and nature, their new story contained no natural limits. It was not multisensory. By the 16th century this disconnected way of thinking worshiped the stories of mechanics and mathematics as pure truth. They validated them as such when Copernicus mathematically proved that the theologian's world view was wrong. He showed that the sun, not Earth, was the center of the solar system. Cartesian and Newtonian stories declared the universe to operate mechanically, to be a non-feeling machine that we could comprehend through the mathematics of physical science.

Today, we continue to learn to know ourselves and the world through tropicmaking stories. They further wrangle and mold our thinking, relationships, and destiny. They and their economics goad us to assault and grind the natural world into indoor tropics. We are not taught that we are each nature, too. Anything that assaults nature, assault us as well. We don't learn that in our detached environment, our thwarted and injured old brain natural senses produce stress, depression, and gnawing dependencies instead of joy. We are wrangled to disown our inner nature, the color of our lives. We create an overdose of G/O stress along with consciousness and environments devoid of nature and G/G. The hurt from our disconnection has led Chellis Glendinning to say she is not in recovery from being assaulted, she is in recovery from Western civilization. We bond to our way of life so strongly that even as the stories change, our emotional ties and the risks of change insanely hold us on an irresponsible course.

Our tropicmaking consciousness emphasizes that, for survival, people must respect, strengthen, and obey tropicmaking reasoning and language. Tropicmaking logic says that these two senses are most attractive for they, not the natural world, are our means to survival. Our leaders teach us to trust them and the useful labels, stories and artifacts they create. We learn that the natural world has abandoned us. It is portrayed as fluctuating and unstable. Tropicmakers feel it is best used as a resource for making our womb-like indoor world.

The tropicmaking story appears reasonable. Historically, it has worked. Our senses of reason and language have registered and internalized it in consciousness and bonded NIAL in us to it. Because we are conditioned to believe that reason and language are most attractive for survival, these two senses became trained, reinforced, and empowered while disconnected from nature.

Like bullies in a playground, reason and language dominate our consciousness. They are a programmed habit that wrangles, usurps, and enslaves multisensual consciousness. Survival by sensing the whole of life is bullied into survival by our reasoning and language abstractly remembering stories that applaud the tropical environment. They comparatively and judgmentally label, measure, subdivide, and manipulate the whole of life, including our screen of consciousness and most other natural senses. Our survival by sensing the whole of life through nature's attractions has become survival by indoor dominated reasoning and stories. The new brain too often disregards billions of years of natural attraction relationships.

The Effects of The Tropicmaking Mentality

Separated from nature and armed with the tropicmaking survival imperative, our tropicmaking reason and language consciousness enslaves most of NIAL within us. It conquers and inhibits the multisensory consciousness which would normally exist. It injures our natural senses. It bonds them dependently to tropicmaking's abstracts and disconnecting ways. Our inner child senses painful abandonment as it is disconnected from its home in nature. It gets support from tropicmaking stories and people when it encourages or engages in nature conquering activities and reasoning. We are wrangled to believe that nature's bounty is for us to possess and exploit.

Although we are in pain, an internal wrangler tells us that our new-brain tropicmaking story is the best road to survival. It still appears reasonable to us. The wrangler contaminates our ability to think with respect to the whole of life. Our natural senses have attached themselves to most aspects of tropicmaking. We fear pain from the remaining sensory bonds being torn from our indoor ways. We feel hurt if a person criticizes our material possessions or lifestyle. Our potential for being hurt because we have learned we are wrong produces barriers of fear. Only our bravest or most foolhardy thoughts and actions hurdle them. Reconnecting with nature activities thoughtfully counter this phenomenon. G/O stress and fear is productively spent as fuel for becoming G/G.

Our indoor learning is not balanced with multisensory outdoor education. Unlike more balanced societies, we learn to disown nature early in life. We find it rude and uncivilized. We seldom seek, enjoy, appreciate, validate, or trust our nature or our natural feelings like we do our money. For example, although only an extremely small percentage of the North American landscape is legally protected from destruction, it has long been against federal law for anyone to destroy a dollar bill.

Like most facets of our society, the field of psychology is a pawn of tropicmaking. Human growth and development research and stages described by investigators like Freud, Erikson, Piaget and Maslow, pertain to helping people survive in our problem-riddled tropicmaking culture. With respect to nature, these disciplines are relatively sterile. They help tranquilize our hurt from our mismanagement of the natural world rather than reconnect with nature. They work well when they include contact with nature's wisdom as an essential component for wellness.

We often don't pay attention to the natural world's callings or to our natural senses. They are desensitized. Our extreme indoor lives seldom contact or exercise them. The natural world is "the environment", "outside" or "nature." It is not us, rather, it is for us to use. For example, rarely does the guide in the nature trust walk, activity 4, have the participant, to whom they are introducing nature, touch or look at the guide's face, yet the guide is nature, too. Predictably, problems result from our mentality's extensive separation from its supportive natural origins and wisdom.

Our disconnective new brain story envelopes us. It urges us to continue to exploit Earth and its people in full knowledge of its detrimental effects. This story injures our natural senses. It renders us unable to feel the emotional pain that would normally redirect us to seek consent from our surroundings. This phenomenon is unknown to other species. When we act destructively with regard to Western people and property, our society calls it war. When we act destructively with regard to nature and nature-centered peoples, we often call it progress. When we recognize that we may sensitively reverse our troubles by using nature-reconnecting activities, our tropicmaking story says we are in some way unreasonable or radical. However, to objectively discover reality, it is reasonable to risk disregarding our story long enough to make a few reconnections with nature and let the experiences speak for themselves. The integrity of this nature-reconnecting process has been proven to bring people to their senses.

The use of nature-reconnecting activities greens our critical thinking so that it values nature. Our fulfilling natural connections with ourselves, others, and the land teach us ecological literacy. We become unified, more responsible, and we feel better. In the truth of the immediate moments of our lives, when we engage ourselves and others in reconnecting activities, we open ourselves to learning from nature and creation. In the brilliance of our 53 sense intelligence, our costly disorders, dependencies, and abusiveness wither. Educationally and therapeutically, the activities support our innate balance of natural loves and spirit. Confidence, self-esteem, and responsible relationships grow from them. What today's immediate moments need are people with the training and wisdom to inject nature-connected learning into themselves and every facet of society. Therein lies balanced living, wellness, and stress management. Laura exemplifies it. She wrote:

> "Reconnecting with nature is about renewing and rejuvenating ourselves to alleviate stress, depression, and anxiety. It uses a hefty dose of fun and great friendships to help accomplish this. I have used the methods and materials on

several levels now, and am beginning to facilitate courses for others taking it. You may be interested in knowing that I am a Type 1 diabetic and have been for 37 years. While I pride myself on my diabetic control, I had for some time been striving to get my A1c tests down under 7.0. This last summer, I was under unusual stress and interrupted my usual therapeutic regimen. However, I had been taking this course for 3 months and doing the activities on a daily basis. When the time came for my quarterly physical exam, I was anxious about Dr. West scolding me for not following the regimen and risking my health. To my surprise, my score was down to 6.1. I firmly believe that by doing the nature- reconnecting activities, my stress and anxiety levels were greatly decreased. I was happier and felt more joy and peace and my overall diabetic control tests reflected this attitude change."

Think about what our world would be if 600 million people in it had daily RWN experiences with nature and their community, experiences that were similar to those of Laura. That thought is the essence of the RWN factor and it is shared by every member of the global life community, no matter what their cultural differences or species. The sense in that thought is the love of life, an essence of Laura and ourselves.

Activity 12: Natural Attractions

Try to feel disturbed about some past or present aspect of your life. Now, go to an attractive natural area. Ask for its permission to become involved with it, gain its consent to help you with this activity.

If the area remains attractive, repeat the activities to register this natural area non-verbally, and then through the word "connection." Now notice that at any given moment some natural connections attract you more than others. This is significant and important. Make your new brain aware of this by labeling each sensory connection attraction. Note the thoughts and feelings generated by doing this. This process gives you permission, (welcomes you to participate) through immediate attraction senses that have often selected themselves on an unconscious level. We are often attracted to what we need, for example, when we feel thirst, we are attracted to water.

As described in the previous chapters, other sensory terms that participants have used to describe natural sensory connection-attractions include: "love," "feeling," "spirit," "sensation," "intuition," "bond," "calling," "resonance," "affinity," "Higher Power," "blessing," "affection," "natural wisdom," "joy," "atmosphere," "God," "sensory fact," "the nameless," "the Tao," "NIAL," etc. Depending upon our upbringing and past experiences, one or more of these sensory connection terms may help identify our experience in green-in-green. Since nature knows the experience without attaching words to it, nameless seems to be another appropriate name. NIAL, the acronym for nameless, intelligent, attraction, love, has proven to work well once understood and experienced through the activities. It contains components that we can experience in the immediate moment. For our society's situation, the words attraction, affinity, or attachment have also worked.

These words describe a cohesive, binding experience, both physically and mentally. They are acceptable in most societies, disciplines, and cultures and safely cross boundaries without triggering arguments.

Some participant's reactions:

"It was as if a cloud lifted off me when I called things attractions."

"I got the same green-in-green feeling from NIAL that I had on the color chart."

"An invisible bond existed between me and the hollow log, "I could sense it like I sense the presence of the forces between two magnets when I hold them near each other."

"Becoming aware of natural attractions is a strong way to feel the connections between myself and nature."

"I felt attracted to the color of the leaf but I did not like its smell so I found another attraction that moment. I was attracted to rubbing it instead and that felt good. It was fuzzy."

Write down the three most important things you learned from this activity and chapter. Write three green in green statements that come from doing this activity. How would you feel about having the ability to feel this G/G taken away? What effect does this activity have on your sense of self-worth?

Chapter Thirteen

The Psychology of Nature Negatives

Nature thrives through affirmatives, attractions we can sense; negativity exists when we don't sense them.

The resiliency of nature's multisensory natural attractions sustains our planet and its life. NIAL has dealt with challenges by transforming them into attractive relationships. Nothing is repelled, or repulsive, so nature produces no garbage. Natural attractions and their collective wisdom insure growth in balance. The source of nature's attractiveness must be very strong.

The news that nature consists of NIAL, a cohesive attraction relationship system, aggravates wranglers within and around us. They subdivide nature into negative stories. Wranglers say that there are many fearful, discomforting negatives in nature. We are warned about hunger, anger, cold, mosquitoes, poison ivy, aggression, slime, bad weather, gravity, snakes, pain, excrement, death, and more. That's why we often avoid nature. Wranglers tell us the same story about our inner nature. That is why we often dislike ourselves. Sometimes, our story takes this nature-disconnected thinking to an extreme. We portray nature as evil. For example, many stories we that we respect assign to Satan the attributes of nature: a tail, horns, scales, fur, claws, cleft hoofs, haunches, and fangs.

A puzzling paradox emerges from the repulsions we perceive in nature. If nature consists of NIAL attraction relationships, then repulsions, negatives, and other discomforts in nature must be attractions, too. The paradox exists because in our nature-separated mentality, our nature-negative sensations and feelings are actually wrangler contaminated stories. To be devoid of garbage, nature must be an all-attraction experience where nothing is repelled. How else can we explain that when we eradicate an "evil" predator, an ecosystem deteriorates rather than improves?

Negative stories about nature result from stories that wrangle us into disconnection from nature. When disconnected, we think with our stories and a few dysfunctional senses. The stories our thinking creates about life and each other are radically different when we are connected to the natural world. When connected to nature, we think in the moment with a congress of multiple attraction intelligences. When we are disconnected, the stories usually don't add up.

With respect to how we feel at any given moment, our inborn natural attractions bring about stability, good feelings, and responsible fulfillments. The wrangler's nature negatives produce uncomfortable feelings and unstabilizing wants. These adverse feelings urge us to reconnect with nature's attraction way of relating. It is important to recognize this because our story of how nature works determines our destiny. It organizes and validates our thinking and relationships. It creates how our lives feel. Nature's intelligence, not disconnecting wranglers, must take charge of our stories so we may build sustainable, enjoyable relationships.

Reconnecting with nature activities help us learn that whenever we sense discomfort in nature, that discomfort is a natural sense, a natural attraction in action. Discomfort indicates that the natural world is supporting us. For example, when we stop breathing or are separated from air, our discomforting suffocation feelings are actually the natural world trying to keep us alive by signaling us to reconnect with air. Suffocation says "connect with the supportive sensory attractions in this moment, seek fulfillment." When we follow our natural attraction to air and breathe again, we return to feeling good.

Nature makes us uncomfortable in order to bring to our attention that it treasures our life as part of all of life. Discomfort signals that something we are doing is out of balance, some other natural attraction senses need to come into play, reconnect us, and provide us with satisfaction. The senses of physical and mental pain play this vital motivational role.

By making us perceive nature negatively, wranglers prevent us from seeing the positive influences of our natural discomforts. For example:

Jim, a course participant, planned to do some nature-connecting activities in the park on Tuesday. He asked me: "What if it is too cold or rainy to go outside and visit the park? What if I am sick?"

"Would that be attractive to you?" I said.

"Probably not, especially not for an extended period of time."

"In nature, as with a hot stove, you risk getting hurt when you choose to let negatives attract you," I replied. "You may reduce that risk by choosing to stay in attractive places or situations, as long as it feels attractive to stay in them."

"So there is value in being chicken?" said Jim.

"Being chicken is just another wrangler story," I responded. "Although your schedule or other pressure wrangles you to go to the park, the weather's discomforts act as a red light and stop you. You then sense a green light from other natural senses such as temperature, reason, place, nurturing and self-esteem. These senses guide you to be reasonable and do the activities closer to an indoor area. There, when you start feeling uncomfortable from the weather, you have a contingency plan at a nearby shelter. That means you have been reasonable which will give you good feelings by fulfilling your sense of reason. If you feel the rainy weather holds some attractions for you, you may discover safe ways to remain outside. Dress warmly, wear a raincoat. Then, fulfilling your attractions to rainy weather will modify your story about the adverse weather conditions. The rain will become fun, an exciting challenge, an attraction rather than an adversity of nature. Going to the park in the rain can feel good."

As we reconnect with nature and validate our experiences, new stories and images appear on our screen of consciousness. Our sense of consciousness begins to know nature as nature knows itself–as many forms of attractions. This allows the new brain to describe nature in loving sensory attraction terms rather than as mechanical cause and effect relationships or as hurtful, repulsive, or dangerous. That is a major shift in our thinking. It results in us learning to enjoy coexistence with nature rather than trying to conquer it. It enables a person to trust building relationships by attractively connecting to Earth rather than remaining mired in the nature-disconnected thinking of our tropicmaking society.

Every natural attraction is a form of love. People did not invent love. We are not the only species or beings that enjoy it. Our new brain can choose to reasonably find love in people and places by validating the old brain and its sensory attractions to nature. That connection is a form of natural love. To choose it rejuvenates and enlists the aid of our natural senses in our quest for love. The choice prevents us from knowing nature as an enemy to be conquered or improved. Instead we learn to recognize Mother Nature, a loving, nurturing parent who knows best about living on Earth because she is that cooperative experience. That experience is the best teacher.

A mother goes to extremes ends to protect and guide her children. Mother Nature does this by creating special senses that greatly increase our motivation to discover and participate in the intelligence of our natural attractions when we don't hear their signals. The various expressions of the natural sense of pain, including mental anguish, play this vital role. If we view senses 25-27 from a nature-separated point of view they appear to be negative, hurtful qualities of nature or punishment for mistakes we have made. However, from nature's point of view, they are wise, supportive contributions. They safely regulate nature's flow like a traffic light. Nature is a vast experience that teaches us to think macro, not micro. In the multisensory macro, pain is a blessing. In the limited sensory micro, it is overwhelming and negative.

When we are fully connected with nature, our story receives the support of many immediate senses. It is balanced. Once we acknowledge this, a discomforting "red light" experience feels more comfortable when we encounter it. For example: the sting of a bee makes us aware to give bees the space and safety they ask. The next time we see a bee we ask its permission to visit. We gain consent and make room for it. We enjoy its presence as well as our presence of mind to keep our lives and its life enjoyable. Said one participant:

> "Because I'm very allergic to bee stings and have almost died from them, I'm extremely afraid of bees. But my natural attraction to the flower's smell, color, and form was so great that for many minutes I was fascinated by gaining consent and watching and hearing a bee not two feet away from my nose. There was no fear. There was an attraction, respect, space and balance that did not frighten the bee. That's a big breakthrough for me."

To summarize: in a nature connected state of being, the sense of pain does not punish us. It signals that we are not in attraction relationships in the moment and calls our attention to fulfilling other immediate attractive choices. It strongly motivates us to consciously decide to move from green-in-orange to green-in-green. It makes us more sensitive to living in the natural fulfillments available in any given moment.

Like all of nature, pain is nameless in nature. In nature-centered psychology, to bring pain into new brain consciousness, we give the following names to the various attraction roles that pain plays:

Physical Pain

When pain's discomfort appears in order to attract us to activities that do not further aggravate an injured part of our body, we call it physical pain.

When pain's discomfort appears in order to reconnect and rejuvenate enervated natural senses, we call it fatigue.

Mental/emotional Pain

When pain's discomfort appears in order to offset, reconnect, or change a story that tells us we will be disconnected from nature's support, we call it fear or anxiety.

When pain's discomfort appears in order to reconnect and rejuvenate us because:

–a story hurts our naturally reasonable thinking, we call it mental anguish. Shame is a form of mental anguish.

–a story says one or more attraction bonds are being denied, we call it anger.

–some of our attraction bonds have actually been disconnected, we call it sadness or grief.

The source of each of these forms of pain is disconnection from nature's intelligent attractions in people and places. The pain may be relieved by doing activities that reconnect us with nature in people and places. In nature-connected moments, our story disappears because nature operates with sensory attractions, not stories.

A feeling of content results from being supportively connected. When we seek nature-disconnected stories, artifacts or people, discontentment is inevitable. The result is a gap in our sensory support and flow.

Negative Stories Affect Our Perceptions

Think about the color chart or the plate of food that had labels saying "poison" or "grasshopper meat" on it. These experiences demonstrate that our old-brain natural attraction senses are modified by our story. We are so addicted to our story that it acts like a pair of colored sunglasses. Once we put them on, we soon get used to it no matter how bizarre they color the world. When out of contact with nature's multisensory reality, we forget that we are wearing glasses that filter and change the reality of what we see or sense. Our ability to cope is limited by our limited contact with many sensory intelligences.

Good reasoning needs accurate information. By the time we reach adolescence, our new brain sees the world through the colored glasses of our tropicmaking nature-separated story. The nature-negative story contaminates our reasoning by giving us tainted information. It leads to our disconnection problems and our abusiveness. Nature reconnecting activities reverse these destructive stories. They safely remove our distorted glasses for short periods of time and reconnect us to NIAL, nature's unadulterated sensory attraction realities. We discover that pain in nature means: "I need to pay attention to additional sensory attraction signals right now." In nature, pain is nature's love trying to support us.

Once we recognize discomforts from nature as being affirmative signals that guide us to overlooked or unavailable attractions in the moment, we place a different image on our screen of consciousness. It asks us to think and relate differently than our indoor conditioning has programmed us to do. It asks the sense of reason to think with natural sensory attractions, rather than with words alone.

This new image does not allow the new brain to scapegoat nature as a fearful negative or dangerous force. To be reasonable, the new brain must see nature as attractive. This honors that nature consists of the attraction relationships that hold everything together. In addition, the new brain learns to honor nature as a beautiful, intelligent, illiteracy; a nonverbal way of knowing that is incapable of acting from a wrangler's story since it neither makes nor understands stories.

Let me share with you two recent examples of nature-connected sensory thinking I recently experienced with respect to negatives:

> At a workshop on a sunny but cold ,windy day, the group decides to meet indoors. I looked around at the landscape and say, "If we go to those rocks up there, we will be warm and comfortable while outdoors." We climb to the rocks and it is as I said. I sensed it would be so because of the direction the rocks faced with respect to the sun (sense #30) and the sense of motion (sense #18). The trees were not moving in the wind by the

rocks. My reasoning sensed we could move to that protected place.

I recently saw *Science News* magazine and felt uncomfortable with the cover photograph of a starry night with a comet in the sky. I investigated what made me uncomfortable. Soon I became aware that in the photograph, the sun was setting on the wrong side of the page (sense #30). The cactus shadows in the photograph were leaning towards the sun rather that away from it. The sun and a sunset evidently had been incorrectly painted on to the night time photograph to make it more visually attractive (sense #1, 45). The sun was shining and the stars were out. This was portrayed as "science" to the public whose deadened senses might not notice the photograph's inaccuracies.

In both these incidents my reasoning made sense of my natural sensory discomfort. We must look further than our stories to enjoy nature's truths. Devoid of input from active natural senses, our new brain lives in a separate reality of its own uprooted and disconnected design.

When we reconnect with nature through multiple natural senses, we discover the difference between what our negative story tells us about nature and what nature tells us. We discover that we may enjoy nature's love by gaining sensory consent for our lives. We achieve this by relating through the immediate moment's attractions to nature. This G/G way of being reverses our negative story about nature, people, and our inner nature, too. It helps us unify in moments that might otherwise place us in conflict with people and places.

In summary: nature is like a sensitive spider's web built of attraction strands. Every attraction strand in nature's interconnected web of sensory wisdom is sensitive to our every disconnection from nature. When we disconnect from nature in some way, each natural sense automatically calls upon other appropriate natural attraction senses to reconnect us to nature. If we disconnect these strands, we become insensitive to these callings and don't respond to them. Then nature wisely intensifies the G/O feeling by increasingly energizing the natural sense of pain. Pain and mental distress reinforce the signal: "For survival, seek and follow the natural attraction that now calls you in this moment. Gain fulfillment, attain connectiveness and stability again." For example, the pain attached to thirst draws our attention to water. It makes water more attractive so we direct our energy to finding water. We reconnect to Earth and its flow of water by drinking. This produces pleasure. Another example: the pain triggered by the sound of thunder may discomfort us enough to be attracted to a safe area and let senses of place, nurturing, sound, and temperature fulfill us. Then we can enjoy the storm.

We may choose to use activities that let us put aside our nature disconnecting stories and open up our natural attraction senses. When we do, we discover that the natural world doesn't cause irritation. It is the wrangling by our nature-disconnect stories and our unfulfilled natural senses that cause our aggravation. When we ask nature to fulfill our natural senses, we gain nature's consent and support to enjoy life rather than fight it.

Recognizing that there are no negatives in nature helps us remove the G/O stories about defects and shortcomings wrongly assigned to the natural world and our inner child. All our inner child knows and wants is multisensory love in order to fulfill it's multiplicity of natural senses. Remember, these include the sense of reason and language. Without stories negating our inner child, we diminish the need to hurtfully conquer it.

Neither nature nor our inner nature is bad or wrong, it is the wranglers, within and without, that impose our nature-disconnected stories that are "wrong". They may be partially "right" for living in our indoor civilization, but they don't contain the wisdom to provide sustainable happiness and life in balance. For example, surveys show that over 75% of the American public are not satisfied with the way they are living. Be we extremely rich or poor, most of us feel like we need 15-20% more money than we have. Very few people feel satisfied with the present or future of their economics, safety, or the health of the environment. Nature-centered thinking suggests that nature itself can provide the satisfaction and wisdom we need. Wise, appropriate stories tell us to choose to reconnect with nature, enjoy it, and grow from it. When we heed these stories, our stress wanes and relationships improve.

In nature, many other senses come into play when we sense discomfort from any one sense. For example, if we feel a strong need for motion or sex or food, the fulfillment and stories from senses of community, compassion, nurturing, space, consciousness, reason, self, aesthetics and many others ordinarily sap the energy from any one sense. This natural ethic prevents any one attraction from becoming destructive. Nature negative stories disconnect us from the opportunity to experience these balancing and supportive natural senses. When these senses are unsupported, injured, or wrangled, excessiveness runs rampant. It has no modifying boundaries from the NIAL callings of other natural senses. That's why nature's wisdom says: "Seek, trust, and heed not just one, but every natural sense that attracts you. In concert, they create wholeness, balance, and multiple sources for support." Without these senses operating, we feel we need our indoor world's laws, dependencies, and wranglers even more. Part of this comes from our conditioned belief that nature contains negatives. We seek a culprit in nature on which to blame discomforting relationships. Our nature-disconnecting wranglers, not nature, are the culprit. We need to enjoy nature reconnecting experiences to obtain new trustable information with which to modify our old story.

The natural world, being built on attraction connections, has no experience in dealing with negatives. This helps explain why negative human stories and behavior are so difficult to curtail. One negative thing or person can often adversely affect hundreds of positives, yet the reverse is seldom true. Our negatives and abusiveness are runaway because they are unknown in nature.

People often argue that negatives do exist in nature. They attempt to prove their point with examples such as "like" poles of magnets repelling each other. Repelling, they claim, is a negative, a repulsion, a pushing away that is found in nature. What their story omits is that their story manipulates the magnet's natural relationships. Their story wrangles the like poles of a magnet together in order to demonstrate that they repel. The story takes the magnets out of their natural state of being to discover their nature and natural state. It leads to false conclusions. Too much of science plays this contorted, nature-disconnected game and leads us further from nature's intelligence.

In their natural state, magnetic substances, like all of nature, exist in attraction relationships with each other. If, perchance, like poles do make contact with each other, what we term as "negative repelling" is actually a force to realign the magnets so that their natural attractions once again unite them. This principal holds true throughout the global life community. Nature's wisdom is to regulate, stabilize, and grow through the beauty of natural attractions. The importance of recognizing this is seen in the following incident:

> At a workshop, Marge came back from an activity with some alarm. She said she found herself attracted to a patch of blackberry bushes. She went over to them and discovered that they were entangled, choking, and fighting each other. That did not feel good. It felt even worse as she did some of our sensory reinforcing activities. They intensified her discomfort rather than her natural attractions. When asked what the blackberries

reminded her of, she said it was like her competitive relationship with her father, "It makes me very uncomfortable."

"When did you notice this discomfort with the bushes?" asked one of her friends. "As I drew closer to them, the details of all this aggravation started showing up." "So if they no longer remained attractive, why did you continue going towards them, why not seek another attraction? Why were you attracted to something unattractive?" said her friend. Marge thought about it a moment and said, "I see now that I had a story that they were attractive and I stayed in the story even though they changed as I got closer to them. Darn, its just like with my father. My story is that I want to visit him because he's my father, so I do, but by the time I get there it does not feel good and the day is ruined."

We soon did another activity and Marge returned from it quite happy. She explained, "I tried not to be, but I was attracted to the blackberry bushes again. It was like a friendly challenge. As I approached them this time I kept asking myself if they remained attractive and why. Suddenly I saw the attractions. The blackberries were not really fighting and strangling each other. That was my story. They were supporting each other so their leaves could get more sunlight and make more space for themselves. They were embracing, not choking, each other. They were a community. They seemed happy, fruitful, and birds and insects were part of their community. The blackberry thorns said to me, 'Don't get too close, find some other attraction, don't interrupt our joy.' That reminded me of how I feel about my friends and this group. It showed me how I would like to relate to my father. I feel great now. Maybe Dad and I can locate our natural attractions to each other, stick with them, discover additional attractions and see what happens. I profusely thanked the blackberries for being what they are and attracting me as they did. That was no accident, I needed them."

Other participant's nature reconnecting reactions to nature negatives have been:

"My thirst actually says, "follow your attractions to water," or "water is calling you." Suffocation does the same thing with respect to air."

"The discomforts from cold, wet weather signaled, "Satisfy your attractions to warmer, drier places. Enjoyably fulfill these callings.""

"The rough surface communicated that I should respect it and protect myself from it. I put on gloves and long pants and as I did, I gained the satisfaction of knowing I was in charge of producing my own comfort."

"The mosquitoes buzz told me to go somewhere else or protect myself if I don't want to be bitten. I appreciated the signal."

"How different this positive way of knowing nature is. It stops me from demeaning or fearing the natural environment as a cold, harsh, dangerous place that I must continuously conquer for comfort and survival."

"This activity makes me believe that every plant and animal lives where it has the least tension and the most support. Otherwise, it achieves this equilibrium by joining some other form of life. No wonder there's no garbage in nature. Everything is alive, everything belongs, everything is attractive."

"I can see how negative people frustrate my natural attractions to them. They have to repel me because their story is that if I get too close, I will hurt their attractions to me, as has happened to them with others in the past."

"The way to relate to nature, within or without, is to only relate through natural attractions."

An effect from having our natural senses injured or numbed is that we have lost our multisensory supportive relationships with the global life community. We have little to fall back on when encountering the tensions from nature's guiding ways. Without an alternative backup, we interpret our discomforts as threats, as nature negatives, rather than as supportive directional signals for survival.

By respecting our desire for multisensory attraction relationships and the supportive community they promote, we discover that our discomfort from:

Loneliness   is really an attraction for responsible sensory relationships.

Depression is an attraction for stronger multisensory satisfaction.

Abandonment   is a strong attraction to being reconnected to a supportive sensory community.

Shame is an attraction to live in a supportive new-brain story.

By safely activating and rejuvenating our natural senses, participation in nature-reconnecting activities reduces loneliness, depression, abandonment, and shame. For example:

> Rita, a quiet, withdrawn person, takes our nature-connecting course by e-mail. She does many of her nature-connecting activities in a grove of large trees in the center of the town square. Through the activities, Rita bonds with the trees. She experiences and validates her strong feelings for them and for the pleasant therapeutic natural sensations they give her. However, the town council designates the tree grove to become a shopping mall and parking lot. The trees are to be removed. Although ordinarily not an activist, Rita feels hurt and outraged by the development plan. These feelings motivate her to act. She participates. She expresses her feelings in every way she can. She talks and writes about her natural attractions and urges others to protect the trees and the beauty they add to town life. Her words and loves of nature activate many dormant natural loves in her neighbors. She becomes more open and expressive. She enjoys supportive relationships with people built on these loves and her inner nature's rejuvenation. In time, she sparks concern in others and they rally to keep the trees. The grove is saved and placed in protection. Through Rita's use of nature-reconnecting activities, the grove has contributed to its own welfare as well as Rita's. Natural attraction sensations triggered Rita's responsiveness and responsibility.

Once again, think about what our world would be like if 600 million people in it had daily RWN experiences with nature and community, experiences that were similar to those of Rita. That thought is the essence of the RWN factor and that thought is not ours alone. In some form that thought is shared by every member of the global life community, no matter what their cultural differences, sex, or species. The sense in that thought is the love of life, an essence of Rita and all the women in the world who have fought not to be dominated by nature-disconnecting stories and those who enact them.

Activity 13: Natural Attractions Feel Good

Learn how to let nature's wisdom reverse your destructive disconnection from being conditioned to tropicmaking and its negative nature stories. Go to an attractive natural area. Thankfully ask for its permission to become involved with it, gain its consent to help you with this activity. If the area remains attractive, repeat activities 10,11, and 12 by knowing this natural area non-verbally, then as a connection and attraction. Now make the following addition: Notice that each time you sense a natural attraction it feels comfortable (enjoyable, good, nice, fun, beautiful, supportive, etc.). Thank it for giving you this priceless sensory gift. Validate this biologic experience and your sensory self by putting it into reasonable (new-brain) words such as: "I am a person who enjoys sensing natural attractions," or "natural attractions make me feel good." Recognize that this validation is G/G. In an environmentally responsible way the new brain produces a reasonable verbal consciousness of enjoyable natural sensations and feelings. This process increases good feelings in relationships with people, too. Some participants' reactions:

"Until now, I never even thought about my good feelings being an invention of, by, and from nature. I just took them for granted."

"In nature, how I feel is just like a traffic light saying stop or go."

"I've always thought these kinds of feelings in nature were a spiritual thing, perhaps they are."

"Thanking my attractions made me feel part of the area, I participated in it."

"When I put the experience into words, I felt it more strongly."

"Validating gave my natural self some self-esteem."

"At the time, I didn't know I was in stress, but I thanked my good feelings for being and I felt relief from something."

"I felt a flow of energy in me, it just crawled up my back and into my head."

Write down the three most important things you learned from this chapter and activity. Write down three G/G statements fashioned from the G/O to G/G information in the appendix. How would you feel about having your ability to create and enjoy this feeling taken away? Does this activity enhance your sense of self-worth?

Chapter Fourteen

The Natural History of Personality

We are each the natural sensitivities that remain alive in us after society has rendered us into indoor people.

Recently a counselor working with cancer patients told me that he found nature reconnecting activities significantly rejuvenated his patients. The problem, he said, was that there were no natural areas near the hospital. Doing the activities was limited to using potted plants and pets. His eyes lit up when I suggested he request the hospital make some of its grounds into a wildlife area that would serve as a nature connecting place for its patients. I also suggested that he enlist some of his patients to help create that area. He thought the administration and some patients would be as excited by the idea as he was.

Our interchange caught the essence of the singular process shared by nature, personality, and wellness. Nature and people support each other. When we participate in the process, we discover a more complete story about who we are and how we relate than is found in most traditional psychologies. This process goes to the source. It lets nature do the work. It incorporates the health of the natural world to replace many nature-disconnected ideas. Our theories are too often stories that try to replace our need for contact with nature. They make us rely on disconnected wranglers and new brain abstracts rather than whole person contacts with natural areas.

Our civilization's weakness is that it does not validate nature's sensory connections in us. It has yet to recognize that the 53 sensory attractions in each of us endow us to live in small, family-like communities that seek and heed nature's attraction callings in people and places. That setting encourages the new brain to help the old brain thoughtfully sense the intelligent ways of the natural world, internally and externally, and translate them into language. Each step we take towards that relationship reduces our rampant problems.

Natural senses and sensory connections are scientific facts. Psychology desperately needs a scientific history of the world that incorporates natural attractiveness. That history would:

-be a developmental ecology of our sensory nature.

-validate that we physically and mentally are a continuum of nature's interconnected flow.

-recognize that the major difference between us and nature is a new brain indoor story that programs our natural senses to attach to the indoor story instead of nature's wisdom.

-show how our nature-disconnecting story prevents important parts of nature from flowing through us due to our separation from nature.

-validate our old brain's feelingful ways of nature-connected knowing.

-confirm our new brain's potential for enjoying and validating the old brain and its sensory unity with nature.

-measure the adverse effects of wranglers and their stories denying our vital connection to nature.

-account for the fact that nature does not produce garbage nor our runaway problems.

-account for the fact that nature produces an optimum of life, diversity, and beauty.

During the moments that we drift out of this history, we drift back into our personal and global troubles.

In many of the natural sciences we observe how nature acts today. We use this observation to explain how, historically, nature acted in the past. For example, as we watch volcanoes shape the landscape today, we reason that past volcanic actions similarly produced ancient landscapes millions of years ago. Those landscapes are some of today's mountains and other geologic formations. Similarly, by scientifically validating our natural attractions, sensations and feelings today, we recognize that these sensory parts of us have been present since their creation during the history of the earth. Our person and personality are living history museums of the world. The list of senses could probably be arranged chronologically and present a history of life. We contain, personify, and continue it.

We have sentiently intertwined with natural life as the following examples postulate:

Sometime in the beginning there came into being a wordless attraction energy. Human beings experience that cohesiveness as a Nameless, Intelligent, Attraction Love (NIAL). A part of all of us was present at that original event and has continued to be present since then. It is our screen of consciousness. Consciousness is attracted to registering attractions and their fulfillments.

Every natural thing contains some level of consciousness and NIAL In reconnecting with nature we enable our new brain to become conscious of NIAL by reasonably identifying it in language as our sense of consciousness or awareness of self.

For any being, the greater the number, strength and diversity of NIAL relationships it enjoys, the greater is its ability to cooperatively exist as itself. The greater also is its ability to enjoy good feelings if it is sensate. You and I enjoy dozens of distinct good feeling sensations that create a powerful network.

Imagine a spider web extended to three dimensions. Picture the universe's growing network of attraction relationships diversely building on itself to look like a web that extends in all directions. Each time a community of attractions finds it attractive to be in a relationship with another community of attractions, it creates another attraction strand of the web by mutual consent. In the process, the network's size and its attractiveness increase. Each attachment strand creates a relationship that provides greater stability for each member of the relationship as well as for the whole web. Like blue and yellow blend to make a new color, green, each new relationship is a unique blending of attractions. It provides a fulfillment that is a fun part of life. Another part of us that was there when it started was our sense of play. We often make connections in nature through recreation, meaning re-creating.

People are part of the attraction web. We experience it in us as the 53 natural senses that play on our screen of consciousness. When we ignore these senses, we fill the void with metaphors and metaphysics that explain the natural world's perfection and how we fit into it. Throughout history, the world has been described through these metaphors such as Indra's net of Jewels, the mechanics of holograms, or the web of life being like strings that attach things to each other. However, to truly know reality, we must experience it. When we experience nature by visiting a natural area, we don't find holograms, strings, nets, jewels, or the like. In nature these stories are replaced by the real thing, by multiple natural sensory attractions and relationships that we can actually sense and feel and thereby register in consciousness. We have too long overlooked these sensations because we spend too little time in nature to validate them. Since we don't live in nature, they have little value. Consider another example of our unreality: one of the astronauts had to travel 250,000 miles to experience Earth to be alive as he viewed it from the moon. He discovered what natural people have always known by being part of Earth through the many senses of NIAL.

Part of us is present whenever new attraction relationships are formed. We know of at least 53 of these attraction modes. They are our diversity of different natural senses. Each is a specific sensory part of our way of knowing ourselves. Each, when energized, appears on our screen of consciousness. Each is a specific sensation or feeling. For example, we feel the appetite for air and then feel comfort when we inhale. We know it more intensely when we don't fulfill it. That disconnection calls up the sense of pain and produces the feeling of suffocation when our connection to air is disrupted. Stop breathing for a while. Check out this reality. Trust and honor your sensation experience. It is an ancient truth. The nameless, ancient, NIAL attraction to air remains alive in us as a distinct intelligent sense. It still generates sensation. In reconnecting with nature, our new brain becomes conscious of it in language by labeling it as a distinct natural sense, our sense of respiration, of re-spiriting.

Each natural sense is part of our way of knowing ourselves. Reconnecting with nature identifies a minimum of 53 sense groups that pervade nature. Each natural sense is an expression and history of the diversifications of NIAL. Each is part of us and also pervades the natural world. Each contributes and is networked to blend with others to produce Earth's intelligent, moral, ethical, all-inclusive way of knowing and being. It makes possible whole system thinking and relating.

Our society seeks, but too often does not find, these natural attributes because we teach ourselves to excessively live indoors. Our nature-separated education disconnects us from full consciousness.

A productive thing we can do is to go through the list of senses while in a natural area and take the time to discover and feel each of them. In doing this we become conscious that each sense is an ancient, uniquely designed spark of life that resides in us and contains a wisdom of life that supports us. The list of senses is like a sensory attachment history book of how nature works through attraction relationships. Often we feel unsupported simply because we are not conscious of the 53 sensory attractions available. A wrangling story overrides them. It says that they, and we, are unsupported and have little value. We feel abandoned because we lose consciousness of our support from NIAL. Our story says our support comes from new brain senses of reasoning and language and the stories and artifacts they create, not from NIAL. We grow up having difficulty discerning if we are worthwhile living beings or cultural objects.

The Flow of Attractions

As it grows and diversifies, the global network of attractions keeps all beings interconnected. Like water or air flowing into, thorough, and out of us, the network lets the different expressions flow throughout so that the love of attractions flows through each natural being. We detect this global flow in ourselves. It lives in us as a distinct sensation. In reconnecting with nature, our new brain becomes conscious of it by labeling it as the natural sense of belonging to a greater being or organism (sense #53). That sense is part of our personality. It is a way of knowing that our indoor lives teach us to block from our consciousness. We often redirect it. We may call it patriotism or product loyalty, an attachment to a new brain story or object instead of to nature.

Nature Centered Community

As attractions grew and diversified, sensitivities were attracted to be in groups with common interests or characteristics that were attracted to each other. They gained consent from the multisensory web to cluster as communities. There are many such examples such as crystals, minerals, species, pods, herds, and societies. Part of us was there when this first happened. That event remains alive in us as a distinct sensation. In reconnecting with nature, our new brain becomes conscious of it by labeling it as the natural sense or sensation of community. It is part of our personality, our way of knowing ourselves. It is found everywhere from microorganism colonies to our consciousness.

Over the eons, our being has become the community of 53 or more forms of attraction that we experience.

Intelligence and Reason

As natural sensitivity attractions built new sensory ways to be, each new sense added additional sensitivities to the global web. Each sense enacts its own special intelligence about life and survival. Each new sense increases diversity as it is added. Nameless nature attractions become more intelligent by being in contact with more and more natural sensory intelligences. The web is a self-governing, growing intelligence in and of itself.

As it matured, it increasingly took the time to balance the different signals from the wide diversity of different senses. This process enabled NIAL to increasingly become more intelligent. We were there while all this happened. The events remain alive in us as the distinct sensation of reason. It is part of our personality, a reasonable way of knowing ourselves.

Billion of years after NIAL became aware of itself as an intelligent way of knowing and being, it actualized through human mentality. The sense of language made it possible for our screen of consciousness to become verbal and literate. The screen became conscious of its own being through a verbal story. Without the story, the screen of consciousness was like an eye. Remember, an eye sees the environment but it can't see itself. That is the consciousness found in most other species. They mostly know themselves and the world as immediate attractions, not verbal stories, and they accordingly relate in balance to each other because every natural attraction speaks for itself. In humanity, through new brain stories, consciousness became conscious of itself and its power as a storied being. Language symbols became abstract shortcuts. They furthered the sense of consciousness by shortening the time needed for the new brain to create a story of how nature worked. People could survive by creating and following an accurate word-image map, a story that helped us gain consent to exist from the community of species. The story on the map said: "Heed and create sensory stories that honor nature's attraction relationships."

The use of the sense of language to identify NIAL remains alive in us. Over time, our new brain confined itself by knowing primarily through the senses of consciousness, reason, and language. These three became our special nature-separated way of knowing and the path to building stories about how to survive in separation from nature. In reconnecting with nature we label this process as our "civilized intelligence." It is disconnected from NIAL.

New brain intelligence and stories connected to old brain attractions to nature are the essence of humanity's nature centered communities and relationships. This bond is the part of our personality that we disconnect as we create our excessive indoor stories, mentality, and lifestyle.

Tropicmaking Community and Stories

Tropicmaker's and industrial society's new brain consciousness produced the false story that its ability to create artificial environments constitutes a higher intelligence than NIAL. That ability is depicted by our focus on ourselves as being the key to our survival. The ego of the new brain imposed and rewarded connections to itself. It created self-aggrandizing, nature-disconnected stories, rather than stories connected to and emanating from nature. Because of this disconnection, we live in two distinct ways of knowing that often disagree with each other. We grow up bonded to the wranglers who impose the new brain's nature-disconnected stories and to the world of artifacts they build. We also grow up learning to assault nature. Our subjugation to human-centered thinking produces sensations of nature-disconnection discomfort that we feel even while we are in the presence of nature. That discomfort produces the stress and pain that fuel our rampant problems.

In reconnecting with nature our new brain sense of reason becomes conscious of our disconnection discomfort and its destructive effects by labeling it as *being in our story*. Being in our story is part of our personality, our civilized way of knowing ourselves. While in a natural area, we have the choice of being in a nature-connected or disconnected frame of mind in any immediate moment. New-brain domination within and around us wrangles us to be in a disconnected story. The process of reconnecting with nature enjoyably interrupts that wrangling. It suggests that it is reasonable for the new brain learn to reconnect and validate that NIAL and the process make sense.

Attachment Bonding

Wrangled by the mold of our nature-disconnected story of conquest, nature within us has no choice but to gain fulfillment indoors or die from sensory deprivation. Separated from nature, we emotionally bond to nature-detached indoor stories and technologic configurations. Our attractions addict us to survival indoors. We feel that we can not survive happily without the artifacts and people we love. We call it this process education when it attaches us to our society's indoor stories, we call it brainwashing when it attaches us to stories we disagree with. Our natural attachment to nature is so strong that when we replace it with a new-brain word we become bonded or addicted to that new-brain contrivance.

Change only occurs freely when two things occur simultaneously. One: our story becomes responsible. Two: responsible attractions are available to fulfill the discomfort of our disconnection from old stories. Indoor education lacks each of these because nature is not present in either. The outdoor reconnecting with nature process contains them. By starting with good feelings and support emanating from attractions in natural areas, the G/O to G/G process catalyzes responsible change.

Our Story World: A Summary

If we validate the vital integrity of NIAL within us and nature, we produce a blueprint that helps explain and resolve our runaway problems. The blueprint shows that we are born as a spectrum of 53 distinct senses, the natural ways of knowing and being. They relish blending with each other upon contact. They are historic sensitive diversifications of, by, and from nature's desire to be in attraction relationships. When the nature-separated stories and acts of wranglers thwart or injure some of these senses, they become less operant until they recover from their injury. We live in fear, the name we give to moments when we sense that we will again be hurt or disconnected. Fear, until it is silenced, means we are under the influence of a wrangler whose story has made us less whole. It makes us act less intelligently.

The blueprint shows that our natural senses are an intelligent continuum that only exists in each immediate moment. We either make time and space to become conscious of our natural senses in the moment, or we miss out on their wisdom. Our detached stories also only exist in the moment. The big difference is that wranglers makes us emotionally bonded to their stories, not to nature. During moments that we fully enter non-languaged contact with nature, our wranglers and stories of the past and future disappear. When we are fully in the moment, we cannot be wrangled by a story because nature contains no stories. Our stories are replaced by the senses of the moment and their wise balance. They signal: "It is reasonable, and therefore feels whole, to become conscious of this safe moment in this natural area. It is a supportive sensory connection with nature in people and places. Learn to trust the sense of how NIAL feels and its meaning." That experience lets the new brain validate that it is reasonable to be connected to nature and feel good responsibly. That story can become a way of life.

Wholeness is multisensory. The blueprint of wholeness serves as a story that gets us out of our trouble. If we cut off our finger, our senses inform us through the sense of pain. Most people have unwittingly cut themselves off from NIAL and are in the confused, painful state of DE-NIAL. The blueprint informs us of this via the sense of reason. It says: "One can't be disconnected from wholeness and expect to think and function normally. Just as it is reasonable to reattach the finger, it is reasonable to reattach to NIAL. Accomplish this through the G/O to G/G process. Let the powerful blending properties of the natural senses pull things together."

The Nature of Personality and Self

The natural role of personality is to make us attractive in order to secure attractive, cooperative connections with people, species, and Earth. Such connections help achieve enjoyable, balanced survival at all levels. Balanced survival always feels good because it is relatively conflict free. It is good for the whole of life as well as the whole individual.

We usually consider personality without recognizing its relationship to the natural world. This will continue until we train our sense of reason to perceive every person as a unique knot of loosely connected, flowing attraction chains. We experience them as the 53 natural sense groups. Each is a diversified expression of NIAL. Each personality knot ties the senses together, uniting the global life stream as a person's sense of self. The person makes the life stream more conscious of its own presence and gives it additional ways of being. The person knot includes the senses of language, reason, and consciousness; it has a conscious, rational literacy of its existence. Our personality strengths and weaknesses result from the amount of support or disconnection each natural sense receives during our lives.

Our personality can be seen as a natural history of our personal sensory relationships. Our enforced separation from and demeaning of the natural world weakens many senses. Our sense of consciousness is only aware of our supported, more vibrant senses. They have the energy to register on the screen of consciousness and they don't carry excessive pain and become subconscious. Although our natural senses may be indoor bonded, they become our special feelings of self. We respond to "Who are you?" with "I am a teacher, a plumber, or a soldier. I am an American, a reader, a Cadillac owner. I am John." We seldom say: "I am an intelligent balance of natural attractions. I am being wrangled by an abusive story of nature conquest."

Our sense of self usually consists of the senses and attachments that play in our consciousness at any given moment. We experience our injured senses as emotional hurt, as pain to be avoided. We attempt to keep them out of consciousness to avoid experiencing their pain. Self changes as environments and situations change. We are different when in safe places versus when we are being assaulted. Our deepest self is the way that we sense and feel NIAL in ourselves. That self senses that we are part of a greater sensory being and are supported by it.

Social Disconnection

When we see disfunctional sensitivities in others, they often irritate us because we, too, are living through the wrangling ordeals that produce such characteristics. Our irritation arises from subconsciously sensing wrangler stories alive and well within us. They can reenact the hurtful incidents, painful abandonment, and inner void that gave us these problems. We try to avoid the potential of having to live through that injury again as we relate to an injured, desensitized person. They often seem threatening and obnoxious until we find our common hurts and desires for reconnection. Often, we can then become strong friends.

Injured senses pass on their injury. An injury to a natural sense results in pain and desensitization. The pain demands fulfillment, often irregardless of the effects. The desensitization results in insensitive disrespect for that same sense in other people. For example, a person with a disfunctional sexual sense may express themselves by sexually assaulting other people. That person has a strong need for fulfillment of their hurt sexual sense. In addition, the victim's sexual hurt falls on deadened sexual sensitivities of the assaulter. This phenomenon blindly passes the original sexual hurt from person to person, generation after generation. Each generation swears they will not hurt their children or others the way they were hurt as children, yet often they can't recognize or responsibly guide their injured, frustrated, desensitized senses and feelings. The hurt part of a person becomes like the hand stifled by being wrapped in a towel. It has to insensitively hit harder to obtain sensation.

Every mentor, therapy, or therapist that achieves responsible results ultimately does so because they have enabled their client's reasoning to more fully reconnect and rejuvenate one or more natural senses. New energies from each rejuvenated sense reeducate internal wranglers. They support and improve a person's total well being and help make space for other injured senses to heal. However, if we attach to the excessively materialistic, exploitative stories of our indoor world, we attach ourselves to the troubles we are trying to avoid. They will appear again in a different setting. They will appear whenever new stress removes the satisfaction that heals old hurts.

Our sensory injuries make us demand more support from the environment than we give in return. For this reason, Earth today is like a sick, worn out mother. She is gasping for fresh air, running a fever, poisoned, and seeking supportive nutrients. As she painfully follows her path, we may sing her praise and pray for her health, welfare, and spirit. What we don't do is change our abusive ways. Our addictive dependency to use natural resources in an unsustainable fashion continues. The secret to personal and social sanity is to learn to be supportive of Mother Earth by connecting ourselves to NIAL in natural areas. That lets nature do what it does best. It helps our wranglers, us, and Earth recover as natural areas gain added value. For example:

Once Sandy validated that she could gain good feelings by following her natural attractions, she made a conscious effort to become fully involved in that process. For years she had shunned walking up the beautiful moss-covered rock faces that called to her in the park. They seemed dangerously steep, wet, and slippery and that wrangling story made them unattractive. But on this day, because she decided that she deserved to have good feelings moment by moment, she followed her immediate attractions to the beckoning beauty of the rocks. She admired their impressive color, height, form, power, endurance, and sparkling texture. Moment by moment she sought and appreciated the most safe and attractive next step across the rocks and, with surprise and elation, easily climbed them. Later, she described her experience and how good it felt. It was now her story. Others enjoyed hearing her tell it and shared in her joy. The rocks had become her friends. She felt attached to them. With her new found support and confidence from knowing how to let her natural attractions guide her, Sandy is learning to accomplish this same result by following her many attractions to better see her friends' inner nature. She is learning how to look past destructive stories and enjoy their soul.

Wouldn't our world be a better place to live if 600 million people had attachment experiences similar to Sandy's? That idea is the essence of RWN. Every culture and species senses the love of life, an essence of Sandy, her friends, and Earth.

Activity 14: Express Appreciation

Nothing in nature is a one-way relationship. As when we breathe, everything in the global life community constantly gives as well as receives. To participate in this process, you give by expressing appreciation to each thing that has given you something. Go to an attractive natural area. Ask for its permission to become involved with it, gain its consent to help you with this activity.

If the area remains attractive, thank it for giving you permission. Did thanking it make a difference? Find a natural attraction there. Now thank the natural thing that attracted you. Thank it for being there for you, for consenting to enrich your moments and for being attractive. Thank your natural sense of language for helping you more fully connect. Thank your sense of reasoning for sensing this appreciation activity as a reasonable thing to do. Thank it for sensing that it is reasonable to feel and express thanks. Thank your natural senses for supportively being there for you. Thank nature for having invented comfortable feelings that lead you in good directions.

Do you feel different when you include expressing your appreciation? Conscientiously asking permission and giving thanks for natural gifts is a good way to sensitize your new brain to things it might ordinarily overlook. It helps open up the new brain to the natural world in people and places. It's how nature works in that everything there both gives and receives to maintain themselves. Some participants' reactions:

"It surprised me to see how thanking my senses and nature increased how good my attractions felt."

"Saying thank you shifted the activity into a whole new frame of reference for me."

"I never thanked a sensation before, but it feels right. For example when I said 'Thank you' to the sensations I had in that lovely bower of trees, my sense of community applauded my sensation of place for being there for me."

"Having to say "thank you" made me realize that I actually do feel thankful for the gifts nature provides. I usually overlook that feeling."

"When I said thank you, I was filled with a warm feeling that was not there before."

"Expressing appreciation intensified the activity for me, it was quite different."

Write down the three most important things you learned from this activity.

Write three green in green statements that come from doing this activity.

What effect does this activity have on your self-worth?

Part Four:
Reconnecting With Nature in Action

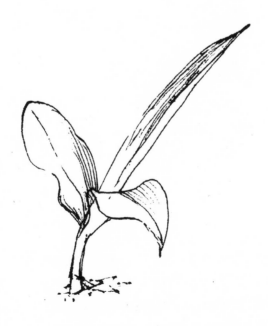

Chapter Fifteen

Outcomes

Most of us are aware that we think with a nature-disconnected process that produced and sustains industrial society. It has unfortunately placed the environment and people at risk. Because our disconnected thinking is missing many natural senses, often it can't make sense of the warning signals we receive. We must learn to use a more sensitive thought process to think our way out of the problems we have thought our way into.

Our underlying problem is the destructive story of industrial society. It teaches us to know nature's love as an enemy. Deep down most of us have learned to fear nature as evil. Our thinking assaults and conquers nature within and around us as we deteriorate our lives and all of life.

Nature's cohesiveness has "wired" us to relate in supportive balance. When people make thoughtful contact with nature, they become more sensitive to life. They build personal, social, and environmental relationships in more enjoyable, caring, and responsible ways. The beauty and integrity of nature inspires them. Their spiritual relationship with the outdoors empowers and guides them. Natural areas nurture them. Contact with nature's cohesiveness has proven to reverse many troubles.

As you read on, you will discover how much the propaganda from our conquest of nature has affected your thinking. You will learn of outcomes already achieved from the use of Applied Ecopsychology and you can decide if they are believable and doable in areas of your life. The following incidents suggest that your happiness, humanity's destiny, and life on Earth as we know it depends on our ability to become involved in reconnecting with nature.

April 18, 1972. Karen, a high school junior, says to her principal: "Dr. Miler, you can't teach me what I want to know because what I want to know is how not to be like you." Karen's words come to mind more and more as I watch well-intentioned folks hurt themselves, each other, and Earth. Their best thinking about how to solve our problems has proven not to be as effective as it needs to be. Karen, after many attempts to "adjust," had decided to drop out of school. She was an excellent student and Dr.

Miler pleaded with her to remain. He pledged that he would teach her anything she wanted to know. That's when she told him that he did not have that ability. She explained that the effects of his thinking depressed her. They showed that neither he nor the faculty knew what she wanted to know, much less how to teach it. That knowledge was seemingly unavailable to the public in 1973. It is, however, available today.

Although they played their role well, Karen's faculty was a typical cross section of society, as teachers are today. For example, 30% of them smoked cigarettes. Because they protected others from the smoke by providing themselves with a smoking area, they were within their legal rights. Smoking was not, and is not, illegal. On the contrary, it is encouraged. Parts of agriculture, industry, advertising, and the government budget depend upon tobacco and its effects to sustain their existence. Karen felt that if cigarettes became illegal, smoking and its adverse effects would not stop. In her social studies paper she wrote "It would be like deer hunting. In some states more deer are poached illegally than are legally killed during hunting season." In that paper Karen also said "We can't make sense of how society educates and governs us because it is not sensible." She was fed up, and she was fed up with being fed up.

Karen discovered what most people already know. With respect to helping us sustain happy, responsible lives, the education we receive is no more effective than the warning label on a pack of cigarettes. Karen was different than many students. In counseling, she learned something extra. She discovered that she wanted and deserved more than what school provided. She began to realize that the world and its people were at risk. Her paper said "We are in jeopardy. We don't just need information, we need a process. We need the community experience to promote personal and global recovery. I want to learn how to build responsible relationships. That is not happening in this school. To teach it or learn it, you must live it. I have tried, in vain, to make that happen here."

At a meeting, the faculty pleaded with Karen to stay in school. "I'm afraid to stay," she said. "The abusiveness in the world scares me." She choked, "We are on the brink of nuclear war. And the natural environment is deteriorating so quickly there may not be a world for me to live in." Her tears flowed freely. "There is nothing abnormal with me feeling depressed at times. The hurt I feel is real. It comes from knowing and watching people or animals being killed. I am tired of putting band-aids on that hurt in counseling and thinking there is something wrong with me personally. That hurt will only disappear as abusiveness disappears and sensitivity, peace, and balance reappear. That is not happening here. This school is contaminated, it's a breeding ground for our problems. It's not healthy for students to learn here."

Mrs. Cook tried to speak. "Let me finish please," Karen said, and continued: "The school has just bulldozed the natural area on the building's west side to build still another lawn. That area was not just a nesting and feeding habitat for birds. It was a womb for all forms of life. It was a place that I loved, where I could find peace at lunch time and after school. Compared to being in class, or even in counseling, that place made sense. It was beautiful, it felt right. I could go there when I felt depressed about my life. I could safely feel all the beauty and life that flourished there. In just a few minutes, I would feel much better. I refuse to be touched by the thinking here that chose to bulldoze that wild area," she said. Dr. Miler interrupted, "Karen, there was no choice. That was part of a legal contract from years ago. We had to fulfill that contract or be sued. And some students smoke marijuana in that area."

"I don't smoke marijuana," said Karen, "I feel sad for those that do. I feel even sadder that the law says that I must spend ½ of my waking life in school. This mentality is bulldozing paradise to make still another lawn. Dr. Miler, you once told me that we learn more from the world around us than we do from books and lectures. I simply refuse to trash paradise or learn to do it. I refuse to let you rub off on me any further. What's wrong with that? It makes sense to me."

She seemed stronger for her statement and its intensity. "Earth and its people are at risk," she said, "Every year in this country, five thousand square miles of nature are being bulldozed into oblivion. How can you possibly teach us to deal with that massacre when you are engaged in it? What are you thinking? What sense is there for me to sit in Social Studies class to discover that our nuclear generating plants are dangerous yet their total electrical output equals the energy this country uses just to run hair dryers? That makes no sense. What do we learn here that helps us stop using hair dryers? To be accepted here, I feel pressured to use one, not to stop. Where is the sense in that? In Biology we learn that two decades ago Rachel Carson showed the danger in using pesticides and chemicals. Since then, we've introduced thousands of new chemicals into the environment every year. What are you thinking when you use these chemicals on our lawns here? I don't want to learn to think like that. What kind of a world are you teaching my mind to build?" she asked passionately.

Dr. Miler calmly advised Karen that the school did the best it could. If she left, she would be truant and there would be consequences. Karen replied: "I don't care. I choose to learn elsewhere. It's too stupid here.

Here, society sentences me to live in an irresponsible mold, an indoor learning environment that assaults the natural foundations of life." This environment is so controlled and stifling that most students are drugged out or into something that is self-destructive or socially harmful. Mrs. Cook, the English teacher, objected, "I, and other faculty members, have taught you repeatedly that these things don't make sense." "Not really," Karen retorted, "You merely say these things don't make sense. What you really teach me by forcing me to be in this unchangeable setting is that I must adopt being part of a runaway stupidity. You don't teach me how to successfully deal with it and I don't want to put up with it. Wake up, Mrs. Cook! You don't know how to stop it so how are you going to teach that? Am I supposed to just accept your belief that the communists and minorities cause our problems? At church we have a conflict as to whether it is right to subdue the Earth as the Bible says. Isn't there a separation between Church and State? You are not compelled to subdue the Earth, so why do you do it and teach it?"

"This has nothing to do with religion" said Mrs. Cook. "Maybe not to you." Karen replied, "That woodland was a cathedral. Weren't the lives of our greatest spiritual leaders shaped by profound experiences in nature?"

Smiling, Mr. Langely, the social studies teacher said: "Karen, cheer up. You are going to be the first woman president of the United States." Wiping her tears, Karen stammered "Oh sure, the first president with a prison record. State laws say I will go to prison if I am truant. That sucks! I don't care, I'll take my chances. Go ahead, turn me in. The law has me jailed here right now anyhow. The big advantage to being in this jail is that I can walk out and find a better way to learn. That's what I'm doing," she stated confidently. The following semester, Karen enrolled in the outdoor school I founded. So did Mr. Langely. The curriculum I designed let contact with nature and nature-centered people teach students of any age how to be more personally, environmentally, and socially responsible. In the process, they learned the academics they needed to meet that goal.

Karen's words bring to mind a study done by a sociologist in Maine. It shows that the students' level of morale in a high school is the same as the prisoners' level of morale in a state penitentiary. My research shows that this does not happen if you teach people techniques that enable their thinking to tap into nature's wisdom.

Was Karen foolish to leave her school? She finished her education through courses that taught the information and activities in this book on how to reconnect with nature. Today, courses and degree programs using it are available through guided home study activities, workshops, and internships. Mr. Langely facilitates some of them. You can learn the process through the activities in this book. Karen went on to become a successful environmental lawyer, professor, and advocate for sustaining responsible relationships.

Most of us grow up not recognizing that in every outdoor natural area, like the wild area next to Karen's school, natural life is not murdering life. It is NIAL, it is nurturing it. The natural world also nurtures and sustains life and diversity without producing garbage, pollution, or insensitive abusiveness. Nature is an unimaginable intelligence that we inherit but suppress.

Leaping forward to the present, we continue to abuse the world and ourselves. As human populations soar, seventy percent of the world's bird populations are declining. Species, genetic integrity, topsoil, potable water, forests, and interpersonal cohesiveness are disappearing at an alarming rate. So are young people with the fortitude of Karen. Runaway stress, greed, violence, crime, diseases, and substance abuse continue to plague us. So do the costs to contain these problems. People have little hope for living in an economically and environmentally sound, safe society. These evils have one thing in common. All of them are unknown in natural areas. Their root is not nature. Their root is our thinking's estrangement from nature's ways. Yet, at any given moment in our life, our every thought, feeling and act, results from the motivating intelligence coming from one or more of our natural senses. In a society hell bent on conquering nature, it is normally taboo to learn or teach that each of us is born with a cohesive multitude of intelligent natural sensitivities that wisely govern nature and our inner nature.

In our society, where can an individual learn that? Education is very structured in our society. In your school, did they teach you how to use nature's multisensory intelligence? Even if we learn about our senses cognitively, it does not mean we will actually feel them. Reciting them is not sensing them. We need to learn how to rejuvenate these senses and bring them back into our consciousness. Then we can think with them. Without them, we will continue to lose our joys, sense of wonder, and responsible relationships.

Our disconnected thinking separates us from nature's reality. For example, we are more in love with pictures taken of Earth from the moon, a quarter million miles away, than we are with the multitude of old brain sensitivities that make tangible contact with Earth.

Despite evidence to the contrary, we believe our present irresponsible way of thinking can sustainably manage our lives and Earth. Can we objectively make sense of our situation if we deprive ourselves of our natural sensory signals and wisdom?

We still learn how to think today as Karen was taught to think more than two decades ago. For example, we still pulverize the area around our home and school into a lawn. We do this even though we know that many lawns require toxic chemicals and that they replace vital wildlife habitat. Nonetheless, our ingrained, nature-separated language story dominates our conscious thinking. That story says:

"Lawns are beautiful;" "we are cleaning up the area;" "it's part of the American dream;" "it is against the town ordinance not to have a lawn;" "a lawn increases my property value," "I'll feel out of place if my place looks different than the neighborhood;" "it gives me a sense of pride." "I've always had a lawn;" "a natural area breeds dangerous things;" "it gives me something to do;" "it provides a safe way for me to be outdoors;" "lawns are our culture and history."

Under this nature-disconnecting barrage of stories, our love for natural areas transforms into a love for lawns. Lawns, and many of our other questionable choices, flourish because our nature-disconnected stories, not the wisdom of our inner nature, shape our thinking.

I know and enjoy the people that made the above statements about lawns. They are wonderful friends socially, but about 85% of their connection to nature has been amputated from their consciousness. They enjoy the natural world through correct symbols and language, not by actual contact. They suffer from our problems because the natural integrity of their lives and sensitivities has been as disintegrated as the natural areas that once thrived where their lawns now exist. Their consciousness is boxed into the limits of our society's indoor world view.

Deep down, each of us sincerely desires to live responsibly in a healthy, safe social and natural environment. But because they are one in the same, as we assault nature around us, we assault nature within us and vice versa. We can not do one without doing the other. My research using reconnecting with nature techniques shows that without using these techniques, we do not have the capacity to teach ourselves what we need to learn and know about living in balance. Like many other products, lawns are not just a choice. They are more often dependencies or addictions that substitute for normal, powerful natural fulfillments from nature. The absence of nature drives us to attach ourselves to fulfillment from artifacts, substances, stories and beliefs, often no matter their adverse effects. Without reconnecting to nature to revitalize and fulfill our natural sensitivities, we remain insensitive to life in people and places. That is how and why we place the world at risk. Ours is not simply a technological or spiritual separation. It is a profound biological and mental disconnection from how nature works within us, globally and perhaps universally. The good news is that our disconnection can be reconnected through sensory nature activities.

Today, as it did 25 years ago, our thinking denies the painfully obvious: we are addicted to our present way of thinking, its limited capacities and disastrous results. With our natural senses missing from consciousness, we do not have the ability to become unaddicted. We can't consciously think sensibly and reverse our personal and global troubles. For our rational new brain to admit this is degrading, so we deny it. It hurts our personal and collective ego to recognize that our nature disconnected reasoning power is far less capable than we say it is. We seldom admit that nature's intelligence manages the world better than we do. A fungus thinks better than us. For example, a fungus, not we, invented the miracle of Penicillin in order for the fungus to sustain a responsible balance with microorganisms. It is easier for us to suppress this painful truth than face it. Nevertheless, even a spoonful of soil contains far more intelligence than we do with respect to responsibly sustaining life in balance. It makes perfect sense to reconnect our nature disconnected thinking with nature's balanced intelligence. Without the higher power available in nature-connected intelligence, how can we recover from our irresponsible ways?

To cope with our senseless disorders, a majority of us are in counseling or recovery programs of some kind. Counseling helps us revive our senses and bring into consciousness deeper thoughts and feelings about ourselves and our relationships. Karen was in counseling long enough to act upon these sensibilities. Have most of us yet learned to do that? Ask yourself: Are you satisfied with your life and its potential? What you think the future holds economically? What is the future with respect to living safely? What future does the environment have? What are the chances of finding healthy, supportive, personal and community relationships? What confidence do you have that we can change the destructive course we presently follow? When I ask these questions of myself and others, I rarely receive positive responses. Most people hold little hope. Over 75% of our population express that they are dissatisfied with their lives right now. Many are in stress and despair. They have been led to believe this indicates that something is wrong with them personally. Something is dreadfully wrong when, no matter how rich or poor they are, people say they need about 20% more income to buy goods, services and security. That dissatisfaction may fuel our economy, but the adverse effects of it further unbalances our budgets, mentality and relationships. It is no accident that the way of life we hold in common produces life out of balance and places the world at risk. Vested interests within and around us sustain our troubles. Many of our inherent natural senses hurt so much that they need things to remain as they are. These senses include feelingful loves for humility (natural sense #40), nurturing (#28), community (#34), place (#30) and trust (#34). Too often, we abuse and injure these and other natural senses. Like refusing to touch a hot stove, these senses won't risk further abuse. As with Karen, when real or imagined situations confront us, our natural senses withdraw, get hurt, or become abusive. Many say that this is human nature. That story further misleads our thinking. Nature is nurturing, not abusive. Things in nature are not abused. They are loved into participation that further contributes to the natural community. That is why nature does not produce our runaway problems and garbage.

On a macro level, nothing in nature is abused, left-out or abandoned. Nature practices a form of unconditional love, not abusiveness. Until we get that message feelingly into our thinking, every time we think we deepen the rut we are in. It is not nature that allows us to assault everything within and around us. It is our thinking that is the source of runaway personal and global abusiveness. Before it was bulldozed, the small natural area by Karen's school was a self-sustaining natural community. It was a showplace for nature's beauty and integrity, an oasis of natural intelligence, peace and global sanity. Who or what was being abused there by nature? It makes no sense to blame nature for the crimes people may have committed in that park. No doubt the abuse of their inner nature was a motivating factor in their crimes. They became desensitized to the life of their victims and their own welfare, too. Our predicament is that this truth is unthinkable in many circles.

Thinking With Nature

Reconnecting with nature activities effectively reverse our destructive separation from nature by scientifically following a proven medical procedure. Excellent medical thinking and research have created surgical techniques that reattach an amputated arm back to the body. If reconnected properly, the arm will, in time, function normally. Part of this art is the surgical technology our thinking has intelligently devised to bring the arm back into proper contact with the body. The remainder of the procedure is the intelligence to trust that once this reconnection is made, only nature itself has the wisdom to heal the rupture and rejoin the arm and body as an integrated organism. We don't know how to achieve this final attachment, however nature does. For example, nature's regenerative ways can, with time, heal a scrape on our knee or bring a bulldozed natural area back to its original state. Good medical science respects nature's regenerative powers. It provides the proper environment and time for nature to heal, as only nature can. The reconnecting with nature process does exactly the same thing with respect to our extremely nature-separated psyche and thinking. Its techniques create potent, nature connected, short periods of time and space in natural areas that lets nature rejuvenate our injured natural senses and lets them create balance.

Because thinking and feeling this way is sensible, fun and feels good, we bond to it. It fulfills our natural senses of play (#29) and reason (#42). It becomes part of us. Have you ever sat near a roaring brook and felt refreshed, been cheered by the vibrant song of a thrush or renewed by a sea breeze? Does a wildflower's fragrance bring you joy, a whale or snow-capped peak charge your senses? Do you like pets, house plants or heart to heart talks; to be hugged and honored by others; to live in a supportive community? You did not take a class to learn to feel these innate joys. We are born with them. As natural beings, that is how we are designed to know life and our life. This book's sensory nature activities culturally support and reinforce those intelligent, feelingful natural relationships. In natural areas, backyard to back country, the activities create thoughtful nature-connected moments. The reader who has been doing them recognizes that in these enjoyable non-language instants our natural attraction senses safely awaken, play and intensify. Additional activities immediately validate and reinforce each natural sensation as it comes into consciousness. Still other activities guide us to speak from these feelings and thereby create nature-connected stories. These stories become part of our conscious thinking. They are as real as $2 + 2 = 4$.

This reconnecting with nature process connects, fulfills and renews our thinking. It enters the natural world's beauty, wisdom and peace into consciousness. The process triggers thinking that values natural sensory relationships with people and places. It empowers us to create stories that are congruent with nature. It regenerates natural connections and community within ourselves and with others and the land. In time, we begin to habitually feel more content, sensitive and responsive. We actively, safely participate in building balanced relationships from this resiliency. We responsibly seek and sustain our feelings of well being. All this we gain from connecting with nature in natural areas and in each other.

Our natural lives have been ruptured by nature disconnected thinking. Although we can sometimes sew up a hole in a ruptured volleyball, we don't know how to repair nature. However, nature knows how to regenerate itself. What we can do is reconnect with nature. The energy generated by reconnecting is like replacing the air that is lost through the volleyball rupture. In nature, replacing that air gives the rupture time to heal itself.

Too often, we choose to live in the fantasy glow of our new brain stories rather than participate in conscious sensory contact with nature and people's nature. The reconnecting with nature process goes a step beyond our stories. Not surprisingly, research shows that participation in nature reconnecting methods and materials is measurably beneficial to people and the environment. In youngsters or adults, participation in them significantly reverses many troubles. It increases creativity, critical thinking and wellness. Environmental literacy, citizenship, and learning ability rise. Participation reduces apathy, abuse of people, substance abuse, depression, sleeplessness and loneliness. We enjoy educational, environmental, aesthetic and economic benefits. Our spirit, energy and self-esteem soars. We actively protect natural areas and help them recover, for they gain added value. When they are abused, we feel the pain and react constructively.

The raw data that supports these results speaks for itself. For example, the article in the appendix describes a study group of apathetic, low self-esteem, depressed, physically and sexually abused, chemically dependent, at-risk students living below the poverty level. They were in a 10 week recovery program that incorporated reconnecting with nature techniques. These youngsters are part of the population that is easily hurt and therefore very resistant to responsible change. The study reports results that are exciting in comparison to a control group that did not use the reconnecting with nature program. Average scores improved dramatically with respect to depression, sleeplessness, self-esteem and stress management. Every student's attendance and academic progress improved as did their environmental awareness, enthusiasm and literacy. No indications of chemical remission were observed 8 months after the program ended. Within 6 months some of the students offered to help the counselors teach the reconnecting process to other students.

Substitutes for seamless nature reconnecting experiences subvert us. Substitutes subconsciously support our delusion that we are intelligent enough to create substitutes, that we don't need nature itself. That delusion is our problem, not its solution. That kind of thinking has brought us to our runaway troubles, not prevented them. To achieve global integrity and balance, I argue that we must reasonably, consciously place our nonverbal sensory inner nature in direct, safe contact with its nurturing source in nature and then speak and live the truth of those experiences. Sanity is nature's intelligence, the nonverbal, regenerative, nurturing powers of natural things and places. When we learn to think, speak and act out that intelligence because it is reasonable to do so, we are sane. We desperately need that sanity today. It is available and it is the hope of tomorrow. That profound, immediate, contact relationship has balanced and sustained nature-centered people and the natural world throughout history. It has shown to work as effectively with our problems now as it did with other challenging problems in other times, places and cultures.

Knowledgeable involvement in the nature-reconnecting process is a vital missing factor in our utopian prophecies, concepts and visions. Too often, we depend upon these stories and government grants rather than get involved with the cohesive process that makes them a reality. We usually take nature's cohesive powers for granted. However, many dedicated activists for environmental and social causes say their actions are motivated by their deep love of life, nature and Earth. Each of us, and every other life form, is born with that love. In most people it has been squelched by the "civilizing" process that teaches us to excessively separate from, exploit and conquer nature including people's inner nature. Our squelched inner hurt fuels most of our runaway disorders, for pain is never satisfied. It is very significant that most adults can not unashamedly say that they love the Earth. That shame produces the apathy that plagues us.

Research shows that you can not simply ask people to love the Earth and, out of that love, act in behalf of life and balanced relationships. The plea seldom produces action. Most people are no longer conscious of that love and its ethic. Without it, apathy prevails. To meet this challenge, the discipline of Applied Ecopsychology enables you to create safe environmental contacts that allow our love for life to rejuvenate and once again be felt. That love integrates ecology. It produces the participation needed to balance personal, environmental and social relationships. If we want to achieve such relationships, it is wise to restore our love for them.

Happily, we have available today what Karen and her faculty did not have available in 1972. Counselor Larry Davis describes it in the appendix B study: "During Dr. Cohen's Project NatureConnect workshop with one of our recovery groups, we visited a damaged natural area next to the student's proposed new school. The area was slated to be paved as a parking lot, and we did the nature reconnecting permission activity there (activity 2). As a result, the student's felt that the area, like themselves, wanted to recover from the abuse it received from society. They sensed that, like them, it had been, in their words: "hurt, molested, invaded and trespassed," "It wanted to become healthy or die," "It felt trashed and overwhelmed," "It had no power, it needed help to recover." Since then, the area and their inner nature has given them permission to enlist the support of social and environmental agencies to save the area from becoming a parking lot. Instead the garbage will be removed and it will recover as an indigenous natural area. It will be nurtured and nurturing, support wildlife, an educational and therapeutic nature sanctuary for the school, and a host for doing these wonderful sensory nature reconnecting activities. The students recently wrote and received a grant to help make this vision of theirs a reality. Here's what they said in the grant's vision statement: "We are a recovery group based on reconnecting with nature. In our recovery efforts, nature plays a major role. We have chosen a small piece of wilderness that reflects us as a community. This wilderness community is being choked by alien plants and stressed by pollution, abandonment and major loss. We too are being choked by drugs and stories that pollute our natural self. We feel abandoned by our society and cut off from nature which fills us with grief. As we remove the garbage, blackberries and ivy we will work on removing the toxins from our lives. As we plant healthy trees we will learn new healthy ways to survive. By protecting this ecosystem we will find the strength to open our minds, hearts, and souls for the survival of our Mother Earth and ourselves." The students in this program have quit using drugs and their mental health test scores show significant improvement. Attendance and academic progress has also improved. Reconnecting With Nature has proven to be a wonderful prevention and restoration tool.

Activity 15 Integrating The Verbal

Go to an attractive natural area. Ask for its permission to become involved with it, gain its consent to help you with this activity.

If the area remains attractive, repeat activity 14, Appreciation. Write or use your previous green-in-green statements This time read them aloud to other people and have them respond to them. Note that you and others feel comfortable reading, writing, and hearing G/G validations. We enjoy seeing or hearing in language (new brain) what is valid and true about our sensory inner nature (old brain natural senses) and their connection to the natural world. That's green in green. Thank people for sharing their G/G statements with you. Thank your new brain for providing good feelings by bringing into languaged consciousness the connections your old brain makes. Now validate your enjoyment. When it feels comfortable and makes sense to you, write and/or say: "It feels good for my new-brain to validate my old-brain's sensory nature and its connective sensitivity to natural attractions," and "I am aware that I gain enjoyment by letting my reasoning-language abilities validate my inner nature and its connections with the natural world." These validations also feel good because they, too, are "green in green." They rejuvenate senses and dissolve wranglers. They integrate our total being, our languaged and non-languaged ways of knowing and being. They also give added values to natural areas.

Some participant's reactions:

"I want to thank Carol for sharing how that attraction felt."

"I feel very connected and warm about this group right now."

"This activity brings nature in people into strong contact with nature in me."

"When I thanked Jim, it felt exactly like it felt when I thanked my attraction to the tree. The similarity in feelings enabled me to sense our oneness."

"At first it felt strange thanking a part of a person's mentality, but I did enjoy what the new brain said and I did feel thankful."

Write down the three most important things you learned from this activity.

Write three green-in-green statements that come from doing this activity.

What effect does this activity have on your sense of self-worth?

Chapter Sixteen

An RWN Activist Speaks His Peace

*Each of our natural senses is a root into the common history
of the natural world and ourselves.*

The following interview with Mike Cohen was conducted by
psychologist Mark Brody and others who reviewed the initial
Reconnecting With Nature manuscript: Linda Copes, Steve Smith, Jan
Goldfield, Gert Braakman, Lorena Tamayo, and Joan Morrison. Numbers
in parentheses refer either to an activity or page that contains an associated
activity.

Mark: Mike, you insist that the natural world is a sensory-attraction
life system that does not communicate with itself in any spoken or written
language. You say that 87% of our mentality that we inherit from nature
is our "old brain," the same ancient, nameless, sensory way of thinking
and knowing that nature uses to sustain life harmoniously. You say only
13% of our mentality actually knows and communicates through reason
and language, our new brain. But the fact is that we live, learn and
communicate in language and reason. What do you see is the cultural
value to us of the old brain, our nameless way of knowing?

Mike: From living in nature for 35 years, I have become sensitized to
reasoning and speaking from the natural sensations that nature has
nurtured in me. That ordinarily would make me a freak of nature, like a
person from another planet whose knowledge has no cultural value in
modern society. However, I have also developed educational methods and
materials that enable anyone to learn this skill from nature. People that
participate in sensory nature activities benefit. The value of old-brain
connecting is that nature's multisensory balance, joy, and wisdom is
missing from our lives. This not only causes our runaway problems, it
prevents us from solving them.

Mark: You are like an apostle knocking of the door and asking people to convert to a different way of relating. Isn't that too radical?

Mike: What's the choice? I know many folks think reconnecting with nature is radical until they do the activities. Then they discover the benefits from the NIAL part of them that they have always felt but could never risk putting into words. In fact, the term radical means that something part of, or proceeding from, a root or base. That describes reconnecting with nature on many levels. The RWN process questions a rooted foundation of industrial society. It says "Embrace nature" while society's roots urge us to conquer nature. We have conquered the natural people and ecosystems of North America. We've separated ourselves from the flow of life. We are out of the loop. Ordinarily, the reconnecting process would be useless in today's world except that it restores a much needed healthy equilibrium between people and with the environment. I would lose my personal self-worth and integrity if I denied my personal experiences and observations while outdoors. People tell me I have been in the woods too long. I find that most of us have not been there long enough.

Linda: What would be your typical day in your nature-connected lifestyle?

Mike: I have painstakingly sought and found some wild acreage adjacent to a tidal bay where I can sleep outside at night, work in a small cabin during the day, and hike or kayak in natural areas as time permits. I'm usually up at 5 AM. I work at writing, participating in the e-mail courses, and public education until about 10 AM. Then I take a nap outside, run up the local mountain and leisurely hike down, experiment with various nature activities, write some more, maybe take another quick nap. Later I may get an opportunity to enjoy my hobby as a traditional singer and contra dance musician. The order of these activities is never the same. I perform as a singer-musician locally once in awhile. Ironically, it is my historical music, not my work, that is utilized by the National Park Service locally. I work as a volunteer for them in reenactments. Sometimes I'm away for as long as a week presenting training workshops and conferences. In the evening, I watch television, folk dance, contra dance, or attend meetings.

Gert: Somehow, watching television doesn't fit your image.

Mike: I find TV alerts me to problems I've avoided by living away from town. That helps focus the activities I develop. I especially love commercials. They challenge me to discover which of my natural senses they are trying to aggravate and then sell me a product to reduce the aggravation. I believe I'm immune to them, but they provide informative entertainment.

Steve: Do you always sleep outside?

Mike: As much as possible, usually in the open under a high tarp without walls or netting. There's a pure natural symphony continually playing out there, a concert of wildlife and weather. My old brain dances to it while my language-reason new brain sleeps. I wake up with fresh ideas that usually enhance nature within and around me. In the morning, I'm putting words to the music I hear at night.

Jan: Does all this outdoor living make you immune to the Western civilization story?

Mike: Not at all. What it does for me is prevent the story from controlling me. I choose to live in voluntary simplicity when possible because I've found that it makes sense in multisensory ways. That's fulfilling so it feels exceptionally good.

Lorena: How did the NatureConnect exercises evolve?

Mike: I originally designed a few of them to introduce my environmental education students to the spectacular outdoor areas we would visit. I let the areas speak through silent sensory solos before we academically subdivided them into discussions, disciplines, topics, and coursework. Later, I realized sensory nature activities could reconstruct the transformative experiences I saw myself and others enjoying in natural areas. I collected and designed many new activities to help anybody have those experiences in their local park, back yard, or natural area.

Gert: What NatureConnect activities do you personally do on a regular basis?

Mike: None formally. I have lived in nature so long that I almost automatically think like the activities work. In that sense, I live them most of the time. The Letting Nature Guide activity is often the way I walk down the mountain.

Mark: What do you view as your unique contribution to the field of ecopsychology?

Mike: My contribution? Probably that I've hung around long enough to see what was going to happen next and try to deal with it. Most of us don't recognize how strongly the reason-language brain is dead set against giving up its vice-like control over our nature-separated lives. It is ego. It has been trained to think we will die if it loses control and we get too close to nature. I offer the simple observation that since our runaway problems stem from our disconnection from nature, it makes sense that directly reconnecting with nature will help resolve them. However, letting tangible conscious contact with nature take the lead, as in activity 17, disturbs leaders who survive by being in control. They want the reason-language brain to invent economically profitable technologies, visualizations, doctrines, schools of psychology, and the like. However, none of these inventions need direct contact with nature to work, so no matter what they preach or teach, they secretly reinforce the story that we don't need nature. Mostly they teach us to continue conquering nature, not to live in sustainable balance with the environment. Making a profit comes first. Nature is dying because our economy thrives by offering artificial replacements for the natural fulfillments and wisdom our natural connections normally provide free of charge.

Linda: What concerns do people have that may inhibit them from wanting to try nature reconnecting activities?

Mike: The activities seem childish and foolish, not profound. They especially read that way. And what rational reason can one ordinarily find to connect with nature? Most people learn to perceive nature as being savage, because nature is a story to them, not an intelligent, supportive sensory reality they can contact or learn to trust. Most of us can spend a wonderful week in the country and still hold to our story that nature is savage or evil. The trouble is that most of us perceive nature-connected people to be native Americans or children, people that we culturally learn to disrespect because they are sensitive and have little power in our society. We are not born disrespecting them. Natural people are not the kind of people who we learn we want to be. Rather we are taught to be winners; to conquer nature, our natural feelings, and others. What we really want to win is good feelings, but they are nature and outwardly taboo.

Gert: Why are we afraid of nature?

Mike: We learn the story that nature is our death rather than the death of our new-brain dominated way of knowing. Infants don't have stories and they don't fear nature. Most of our fears come from our experiences, from new brain stories assaulting our feelings and multisensory old brain. We fear becoming too feelingful or free for it risks getting hurt by the childhood stories we carry of good or bad, right or wrong. For example, as adults we live out the fears instilled by the likes of Little Red Riding Hood, yet most of us have never seen a wolf, nor do I know of any cases of wolves hurting people. What frightens us and annihilates wolves is the "story", the domain of the new brain. If we learn to question our stories or take our lead from nature, the new brain senses it is going to lose its control. We can't get out of the rut we are in because we always communicate with other new brains that agree that new brains know best. We constantly feed on the source of our disconnectedness.

Joan: How should we deal with the current environmental backlash?

Mike: I don't believe we can because its a new brain power and control conflict. Nature alone knows how to deal with the backlash through the RWN factor. When people's inner nature becomes alarmed, it will make its discontent known. What we need is education that supports conscious contact with the nameless.

Joan: Are you saying that the Reconnecting With Nature factor is an initiative by nature to awaken human consciousness? Could you give us a couple more examples of how this process works.

Mike: RWN is not an initiative by nature. It is my new brain expressing that it is reasonable to let nature's wisdom enter and help balance our runaway relationships. The RWN factor simply asks the new brain to be reasonable and make space to let the wisdom of natural senses and feelings contribute to our lives. When that occurs we unleash the supportive natural love that makes the whole world kin. For example, think back to 1988 when two whales accidentally got stuck in the Arctic ice. They would die without help. They triggered a billion dollar rescue effort and media blitz that opened unheard of avenues of cooperation and unity. The whale's sad plight went right through the iron curtain and the walls separating environmentalists and industry as well as science and spirit. Applying the RWN factor triggers that reaction because it is both old brain and new brain sensible for us to support nature personally, locally, and globally.

Steve: If you had a role in our government, what changes would you make and how would you convince people that the changes were economically feasible?

Mike: The RWN factor is a free, powerful, ecologically sound stress management process. A huge portion of our taxes go to paying for the damage done by stress from the conflicting nature-conquering stories of nations and individuals. If government encouraged people to use nature-centered activities to relieve stress, it would create a healthy mental and environmental climate with healthy budgets and relationships to match. The insurance industry could save billions of dollars by promoting it and the public would benefit, too.

Jan: What disappoints you the most in our present political climate?

Mike: Our nature-disconnected political climate doesn't disappoint me. I expect it to be what it is. We elect to office those who best represent us, those who use nature-disconnected language and reason to convince us to vote for them. We reap the rewards of their nature conquering new brains in office. It makes perfect sense, why should I be disappointed? It's no different than electing highly competent people to lead the KKK. You would end up with a well organized, socially supported runaway nightmare. Street gangs serve as another good example. This won't change until we let the wisdom of old brain nature connections guide us. The nameless world best knows how cooperative multisensory survival works because it is it. Our politicians managing the natural world is similar to a lobster running the control tower at O'Hare International Airport.

Mark: Why have all the major religions failed in their response to the environmental crisis?

Mike: They, and most of the less popular religions too, are indoor institutions that revere the dogma of new brain stories, not guidance from tangible sensory connections with NIAL outdoors.

Steve: Can you find the same higher power indoors vs. outdoors? For example, how would you account for people who report profound mystical experiences that feel connections with the power of nature, but that happen indoors?

Mike: Mystical experiences are mysterious because we have no story that explains them. I don't know nature to be a mystical experience. I know it as beautiful, stimulating multisensory feelings. If my senses and feelings had no rational explanation, nature could be mystical to me, indoors or outdoors. Even on our e-mail course, I find that people feel strange when, having been alive for decades, they first experience some of the natural senses that have been buried alive within them. To them it is mystical, to me it is delightful because I know it will happen and I don't question it. I don't trust higher power that comes only from contact with our inner being. It seems limited in comparison to tangible, sensory, non-verbal contact with natural areas. Our inner sensory being has been hidden behind our new brain stories and has been emotionally bonded to our indoor world. Is it reasonable to expect to find reliable support from connecting with an injured, buried part of ourself that has been victimized, abused, and conquered in our war against nature?

Mark: Are you saying that nature doesn't touch us indoors?

Mike: No person is an island. There is natural love in natural areas that touches people and that is missing indoors if for no other reason than "indoors" is the result of a story, not nature's balanced intelligences in action. Nowhere in nature have I found anything natural to exist detached from its bonds to the global life community. I find that indoors my natural senses are not directly connected to nature. They instead connect to walls, images and visions, the story world. Those stories can't deal with nature. Actually, they often exist to celebrate our new brain's ability to conquer. They block out nature. To apply them to our inner nature experience would produce mysteries, don't you think? For example, taking drugs and having an a hallucination of a beautiful forest experience indoors is not connecting to nature, even though that might be what the experience says it is. This would be merely feeling good by freeing up one's natural senses artificially and then wondering why they are there. That's different than doing nature reconnecting for a week and letting nature itself love your natural senses into consciousness and support them. That's ecstasy, not mystery.

Lorena: How would you revise our educational systems?

Mike: I would make the potential of nature-reconnecting education widely known, supported, and used in conjunction with all subjects and classes. That is easily possible through the Internet. It is appropriate for most disciplines. I would insist that its use be encouraged where and when individuals or groups of people want to participate in it. Dramatically, the results would speak for themselves so others would be attracted to participating in nature reconnecting experiences. Over 85% of the public is environmentally concerned and stressed out as well. They deserve and, if supported, would jump at the chance to let nature's wisdom relieve them of the costly stressful economics and hypocrisy that their stories inflict upon them and the environment. The major challenge to education is for it to recognize and deal with the fact that we are emotionally bonded and addicted to our false stories. We need re-education, a process that will safely un-bond us from our present stories and re-bond us to living responsibly. I find that sensory contact with nature has the power to do this.

Linda: What would you view as any sign of hope for our planet?

Mike: Whenever, wherever people learn to relate by enjoying and sharing nature's love, peace, and wisdom within and around them, there is hope.

Mark: What are some key points for a therapist to remember in using a nature reconnection approach with individuals in counseling?

Mike: Two points come to mind. The therapist must be experienced with the G/O to G/G process and understand and trust it. They must let nature, not their personal stories or psychological theories, take the lead. Every time we put a word on our nameless attraction relationships, we risk being subject to the nature-separated dogma that might incorporate that word. If nature, even in the minimal form of a potted plant, is not a key factor in their work, therapists are probably playing God without God's wisdom.

Jan: From a psychological theoretical point of view, how does your approach compare to others?

Mike: My view openly admits that the Western new brain has been deeply contaminated by excessive sensory disconnection from its biological life support system in the old brain and nature. My approach says that psychologically, the wisest thing I or anybody else can do is make space to tangibly, consciously reconnect with nature and let NIAL do the healing because nature knows how to heal itself. This gives a new added value to natural systems, one that demands that they can recover so that we can recover with them.

Jan: Why do you call that a psychology?

Mike: Nature connecting activities automatically bring to consciousness some of the important ideas of psychology. They include the Rogerian model of unconditional positive regard for all, including the self and especially nature, and it is encouraged through the use of attractions. Cognitive behavioral principles are the behavioral component of doing the activities leading to a positive shift in attitudes about nature. This is reinforced in expressed cognitions through the sharing of experiences from doing activities. This is a vital component. Social learning theory poses that much of our behavior, whether negative or positive, is learned from models. In this work, nature itself is a role model.

While I believe that different theories of psychology offer valuable insights, most neglect nature. The theories seldom recognize that they exist as Band-Aids for our separation from nature, that without including reconnecting with nature they might actually be supporting our continued separation. Before I'd trust any other approach, I'd want to see the long term effects of that approach on Earth and its people. What is the use of learning to feel comfortable with destroying your own life support system? With today's knowledge that the environment is on the brink, knowingly engaging in activities or theories whose process continues to let us remain separate from our environment defines insanity. It tears us apart emotionally. Each moment we engage in such activities, the deeper is our bewilderment and pain. The economic issue is not even a question. There is a tremendous economy sitting before our eyes in becoming healers of each other and our planet. The many savings and rewards of doing so could gracefully replace the expensive technological fixes we are now addicted to.

Gert: There are many nature oriented healing practices that have been in existence for thousands of years. Which ones influenced you the most?

Mike: No offense, but none of them, not one. I'm ignorant of them. I was not raised in them as a child, and my adult years in natural areas I've had understandably little contact with them. The few I have seen seem to be stories with human therapeutic effects, but don't tangibly depend upon or involve nature. What little I have learned, I learned from the nurturing and kindness of Eleanor Roosevelt and the educational processes of John Dewey as they apply directly to conscious contact with nature in people and places. I know that Earth can and will teach if one creates moments that let it do so. I also know we are daily trashing that beautiful relationship and opportunity, an ultimate madness. My methods and materials empower anybody of any age to let Earth teach them balance and integrity moment by moment. After all, to engage in this process all one needs to do is gain consent to participate in it from nature in themselves, others, or the environment.

Mark: Why do we stay in the vicious circle of hurting the environment and ourselves?

Mike: Times have changed, but our stories and practices have not. We have become attached to them as is. For example: the behavior of burying our waste may have been fine when the waste was all natural; that practice produced a fertile area as well as a fertile cultural identity. Today, attachments to the same story and ritual may still feel comfortable and culturally essential, but enacting it produces a chemically toxic garbage dump that contaminates water and undermines ecosystems. With Earth's natural systems on the brink, we need to create stories and rituals as if nature mattered. Nature reconnecting activities have well served that purpose for some people.

Lorena: Are there any indoor stories that you trust?

Mike: As far as indoor stories are concerned, I trust the Lorax. I think nature reconnecting activities are the seed the Lorax left for the next generation. A seed does not contain stories. It contains the natural sensory attractions of the eons that produce the wisdom of nature's beauty and balance. It contains the ability to grow and sustain them. Do you realize that most young people today have never heard of the Lorax? We have effectively removed the truth of the Lorax from the story of our central culture. Our story world is so removed from nature that today intellectuals validate our attachments to nature through the research and theories of E.O.Wilson, a Harvard Professor who at this late date hypothesizes that humans have a biologically based need to affiliate with the natural living world. I believe that 30 years ago that need was well established by the sadness that the disconnections Dr. Seuss and the Lorax story fostered. Sadness results from the breaking of intact sensory bonds.

Steve: How can transitioning from G/O to G/G help with feelings of worry, sadness, and depression?

Mike: I think Linda can answer that better than I can. Linda?

Linda: In the past, I suffered from severe anxiety attacks, and at times am still prone to feelings of intense stress. In my experience, these profoundly anxious or stressful feelings disconnect us from our inherent natural senses of support, safety, love, and peace. Using the nature-reconnecting activities positively reconnects us with these senses and feelings. They also foster a sense of nurturing calmness, emotional stability, well-being, trust, empowerment, and self-esteem. The very senses and feelings that are stripped from anxiety attack sufferers are re-awakened and re-enforced by using these nature connecting activities with others. As Nature safely teaches us what is "real" in ourselves, we can gradually replace our "unreal" fears and anxieties with feelings of in-the-moment joy, radiant good health, fun, laughter, self-balance, and harmony with life.

Jan: Linda, how do the activities do that for you?

Linda: They have taught me that nature exists only in the moment, and by doing the activities, and learning to let Earth teach me her wisdom and profound intelligence. I have been able to realize that very often sadness and depression are the result of a "story" that I am reliving from the past. Worry and fear are often the result of a "story" of what might happen to me in the future. Nature has taught me that life is moment to moment attraction forces simply following a "desire to be," and if I can allow my inner nature to exist just as the rest of nature does, then I am also able to intelligently live moment to moment, which releases me from the "stories" of past or future. Hence, I no longer have to suffer from the sadness, worry, or depression. The connecting activities can supportively teach us how to recognize our "story," and how to find and follow our immediate natural attractions.

Mark: Mike, many people in this country are finding their nature connection by studying with Native American teachers. Why do you say that we also need different rituals for our time and situation?

Mike: I haven't had any Native American teachers so I can't respond. I do know from discussions with natural people that the ceremonies I have attended with them have had an entirely different meaning to me and other Western people than they did to the natural people who performed and attended them. In general, I trust a person who is living and teaching a nature-connected life, one that is actually bringing back the natural environment, not just talking stories about doing it.

Mark: Mike, thank you for this interview and for helping to make reconnections with nature happen for me. Each of us here knows that reconnecting with nature is not unrealistic for we have experienced the process and its benefits. The big RWN factor challenge for me is how to describe reconnecting with nature to others and make it understandable.

Mike: It's not possible for words to fully describe relationships built on non-language sensory attractions. My latest attempt is to use an anecdote that Carol says is accurate. You might want to make it part of this interview.

"Carol applies the RWN factor by participating in a nature-connecting e-mail course, whose members live in many different countries. She reads her training manual to learn what G/O to G/G activity she and her e-mail, telephone and local partners will do this day. As Carol begins this day's activity, spontaneously, the delicate sparkle of a water droplet on a fern attracts her. She does additional activities that reinforce this attractive nature-connected sensation and she becomes aware of other times she has felt it. She also notes her past disconnections from it and the effects of the loss. Carol shares her thoughts and feelings from her experiences with her partner in the park and then her 7-person e-mail group. She reads and responds to her group's and instructor's posted nature experiences, and to their response to her reactions. It's fun. She plays the role of teacher, student and counselor. She feels alive and spirited, supported by her partners and connections to Earth. Her day brighter, Carol looks forward to further connecting with the people and natural places that attract her at home, work, school, and in the community. They now mean more so she treasures them and she finds new self-worth and fun in life. Because she has done the activities and known their effects, she owns them and the joys they can bring. She intends to form a local nature reconnecting training and support group so that she can spend more time in sensible community."

Mark: I think each of us here feel more hopeful since we have seen and experienced the value of the RWN factor as portrayed in this description of Carol. Thanks again.

Activity 16: Respecting Natural Attractions

Go to an attractive natural area. Ask for its permission to become involved with it, gain its consent to help you with this activity.

If the area remains attractive, thank it and go to a few objects or aspects of nature one at a time. For one minute, take hold of each object and pull on it, but do not remove it from the attraction relationships and attachments it presently enjoys. Be sure to leave it as you found it. Note what thoughts and feelings come to mind during the minute you are in this balanced relationship with each of the natural objects. Some participants' reactions:

"I felt the seaweed was pulling back, like it was signaling how forceful I should be in order to have both of us survive."

"The Dandelion told me it wanted to stay where it is."

"I felt the blade of grass drawing me into itself and Earth."

"I disconnected the twig accidentally and felt sad."

"This was a real challenge to do with water. Some of it wanted to be with me so my hand stayed wet."

"My hands felt like they melted and streamed into mixing with the flower. My body started to join them. I fantasized we were some natural thing dancing by itself."

Write down the three most important things you learned from this activity.

Write three green-in-green statements that come from doing this activity.

How would you feel about having your ability to create and enjoy this G/G feeling taken away?

What effect does this activity have on your sense of self-worth?

Chapter Seventeen

Self, Meet Yourself

The characteristics of a person and Earth are so identical that one might suspect Earth to be sentient.

The way we are wrangled to think in industrial society makes each of us a god. Only our new brain has the power to imagine a disconnected story on our screen of consciousness and then transfer that story onto the face of our planet and people. Every other species survives through the cooperative consent of their environment rather than through disconnected dominating stories.

Disconnected from nature's flow, we think up our runaway technological world along with its troubles. One way to act reasonably is to use our power of imagination to help us reconnect our thinking with the wisdom of the global life community. Our new brain becomes more consenting to make sensory connections with Earth when it recognizes Earth acts like a sensory, reasonable, living being. To this end, I offer your power of imagination the following guided journey.

Do this 45-60 minute activity in a natural area, when possible. Go on to each new paragraph only after you savor each paragraph you read.

If possible, go to a natural place that includes a large scenic area. Now, in your imagination, sense and feel your personal nameless, intelligent, attraction love (NIAL) and then become it. Imagine trickling down cracks and fissures in Earth's surface. Go deeper and deeper towards the middle until you situate yourself in the center of the nucleus of an atom in the heart of Earth. Now slowly expand into yourself into the global network of sensory attractions that attach that nucleus to itself,...its atom....its surrounding atoms.... Expand yourself along these attractions as you sense them, becoming larger and larger, filling up Earth, becoming all of Earth, including its atmosphere... You are a 10,000 mile thick nameless global being held together by NIAL. You are all of Earth...

Sense yourself. Give your new brain permission to learn from your human life about the planet's life and vice versa. As time permits, find an example in nature for each of the following paragraphs during or after this imagery...

Sense yourself as a feeling, an attractive intelligent desire to relate through attractions. You are rewarded by each relationship's greater stability and gratification...

Let your hands touch each other, and then your face. By reasonable affinity sensations like touching, tasting, thirst and hearing, not by words, do you, Earth, know yourself and survive...

Feel yourself as an intelligent symphony consisting of infinite numbers of interconnected attractions interacting, attaching, and building over the eons...

Press your hands on your temples and enjoy sensing your heartbeat. That pulsating tension-relaxation essence of your life still beats as it has since your birth billions of years ago...

Welcome the sun's presence. Inhale sunlight and feel good about creating oxygen from it. Let yourself hear and feel your breathing. Thank your planetary breath for being, for circulating air through plants, animals, water, and minerals, making their lives and your life possible...

Feel the sun becoming warmer and retain your cool by sweating thunderstorms and hurricanes. Imagine fanning yourself with Arctic air or cooling off with an Arctic ice-water bath...

Feel great about erecting an umbrella of clouds or an array of sunshine reflectors made of daisies, snow, or glaciers...

Feel hungry and satiate your hunger with sunshine...

Sense your lips drying. Sprinkle them with rain to make them feel moist...

Put your arms around yourself. Savor being embraced by the universe and yourself...

Feel relieved that you have organ systems satisfying your need to excrete. Compliment yourself for discovering how to recycle your excretions into healthy food and water that are safely re-used. Feel proud of that achievement..

Relish your sexuality, your planetary attraction for life to continue. Applaud yourself for being a fertilized, growing egg, of the universe...

Feel an overabundance of saliva in your mouth. Swallow it like the planet swallows carbon, salt, and methane to regulate the levels necessary for life's maintenance...

Luxuriate in the harmony within you and knowing how to maintain it by altering yourself continuously...

Honor yourself as a womb of life; feel the excitement of an expectant parent as each new life begins...

Revel in the gratification of inner and outer companionship, a sense of place, support, and belonging; a sense of being whole and important for life's existence...

Celebrate being something very worthwhile. Rejoice that your survival attractions validate all your natural processes; you are never bad, negative, or evil...

Feel nurtured and nurturing. Feel musically harmonic like a simple folk song or a symphony. Enjoy your music as natural sounds, including silence, thunder, and a chickadee chirp. Hum the note that you feel you are now.

Feel wonderful that you are conscious to enjoy all these aspects of your survival. Be happy you are them. Delight in their consciousness of you, their consent for your benevolence, leadership, and wisdom...

Feel secure that even as you sleep, the life process maintains itself in celebration of you...

Resonate in the joy of creating new organisms and life systems that share, support, and enjoy your life and enrich life for others...

Honor yourself for brilliantly establishing life over the ages without using written words, numbers, machines, or money...

Revere your ability to heal yourself when you are injured or under civilization's stress and tension...

Feel ecstatic because you consist of ever-adjusting attraction relationships that release tension...

Revel in looking out into the stars and sensing the wonder of looking deep into yourself and your attractive beginnings...

Cheer being mostly illiterate and not subject to disconnective stories...

Thank creation for having created your enchanted life and potential for enjoyment...

Welcome the delight of your essence. Exhale and don't breathe. As you hold your breath and the discomforting tension builds, know that you are experiencing your global survival voice, a sensory language that knows no words. Celebrate that it tells you to seek comforting attractions now and reconnect to them. Feel safe knowing that beyond yourself is an attraction force that loves you, that reveres your importance, that insists you breathe even if your "story" tells you not to. Now inhale and feel the delight of releasing tension, of reconnecting to your integrity by breathing...

Appreciate that you breathe both air and sunlight...

Feel powerfully confident knowing that your universal attachment language of tension building and tension release communicates growth and survival for every single entity in your global life community...

Appreciate that the good feelings you get from acting at one with yourself express the global community's consent and thanks for you to be in the next moment...

Feel exhilarated by the pulsating signals between yourself and the moon, sun, and universe. Enjoy the tickling of your tides, the streaming of your rocks, the volume of your volcanic burps...

Feel honored and cherished that your survival is the basic origin and purpose of the thousands of differing human cultures...

Love life, because you are life...

Relish feeling unity as you enjoy all the matter and forces of yourself that are manifestations of your attraction to be alive...

Feel the pleasure of unconditional companionship, that whatever happens to you as the planet, also happens to you as a person and vice versa. Other than your human ability to know language, you and Earth are identical...

Adore that as a living organism you maintain your life by relating to the surrounding solar system and universe. Feel gratification as your being flows and bends with its fluctuations and forces...

Feel the bliss of yourself as a global organ community exactly like your human organ community. Hold in esteem that counterparts of your kidneys, liver, pores, stomach and heart exist in your geography. Delight that habitats function not only as homes for their creatures, but also to sustain your global life attractions...

Cherish how your metabolism is driven by ingesting the sun's high energy radiation and excreting low energy...

Feel wonderful that your ocean's kidney is the activity of the continents, oceans, and corals. Welcome their attachments to each other in warm, shallow, inland seas that evaporate water into the atmosphere and crystallize out excessive salts and sediments.

Thank glacial melt and rivers for helping to stabilize your salinity...

Appreciate the tropical rain forests and phytoplankton for acting as lungs to respirate and convert carbon dioxide to oxygen...

Value that continents and ocean sediments are your liver and store minerals that nurture you...

Savor your circulatory system of oceanic and atmospheric currents, of rain and rivers. Delight that they distribute your nutrients and help regulate your temperature...

Hold in esteem your digestive system's love to erode rock with lichens, wind, and glaciers...

Indulge in the beauty and color of deserts, volcanoes, and clouds. They are the skin, pores, and blush of your skin.

Savor the purity of the solar wind plasma and lymph that bathes you...

Rejoice your rotation causing the heart-pumping action of daytime and nighttime temperatures. Feel in awe that your angle to the sun and your orbit around it creates seasons, polar ice caps, and equatorial tropics. Feel the pleasure of heat differentials producing your circulation externally and internally...

Feel the bliss of your musculature, your flowing inner core and continental movements...

Be proud of your skeletal system of continents, mantle, and mountains...

Thank your beaches for acting like fingernails, protecting your fragile coastal lands from wind and wave...

Appreciate your skin-healing scars and scabs, your hardened volcanic plugs and lava flows...

Enjoy your mental energy's networked nervous system of electrical, hormonal, gravitational, and magnetic attractions. Celebrate its interlocking, fluctuating, community sensory signals that interconnect all aspects of yourself...

Delight in your forests of hair that insulate and protect your body...

Feel the glaciers as molars grinding rocks to dust which the wind spreads to make fertile soil to feed the planet.

Trust your endocrine systems of climate and weather patterns which balance hot and dry, wet and cold...

Feel the pleasure of your oceanic rifts regulating your temperature and salinity as they alter the size and place of your heat-collecting oceans...

Relish your breath of five thousand miles of layered atmospheric and stratospheric gases. Appreciate how they cope with the solar wind and universe for you and the plants, animals, and minerals that live in you, not on you...that are you....

Revere your spirit's desire to relate beneficially to every entity of your being...

Feel secure in your wisdom of billions of years of knowledge and relationships of your parts as their attractions perpetuate and regenerate you.

Thank each of the 53 natural senses for the sensible guidance they offer and the good feelings they give you when they are fulfilled...

Savor people as an embodiment of you, feel the pleasure of being more conscious of yourself through their symbols, images and language. Appreciate doing that right now as you read...

Be ecstatic that your consciousness makes you aware of the feelingful callings of your global life system's ways for your survival. Thank your sense of consciousness for cooperatively growing with the life community...

Honor the global community for consenting to your being. In return, give it the priceless gift of your consent for its being...

Enjoy that you were naturally intelligent enough to invent good feelings so that you know when you are supporting the global life community because it feels good...

As a final image, fly out from the Earth, look back and celebrate our planet as the womb of life as we know it. Look closely, and mixed in with its flowing placental clouds, continents, and waters, you will see your adult self, safe and secure. Rejoice that you, others, and Earth still share the same NIAL heartbeat. As we touch Earth, we touch each other. Thank that image and thank its good feelings for being there for you.

Activity 17: Nature as Guide

As in this chapter, Earth itself can be your guide. Go to a large attractive natural area that you can walk through. Ask for its permission to become involved with it, gain its consent to help you with this activity. If the area remains attractive, thank it and learn to let Earth guide you. Safely trust its attractiveness. For eons it has shown that it knows how to harmoniously build community and beauty.

This activity asks your new brain to open to this natural area's callings by following the natural attractions there that spontaneously attract you, rather than by seeking attractions you expect to find there. Your new-brain choice to do this is critical. It takes a risk. It thoughtfully, respectfully, permits and enables nature within and without to take the lead, to momentarily guide you. That is natural wisdom in action, how nature works. This process naturally connects your new-brain with immediate callings from Earth to your inner nature's sentient attractions and desire to be part of nature. Thank it for doing that. This process is not a surrender. In the light of the troubles emanating from our excessive separation from nature's workings, it is a reasonable, intelligent new-brain act. You mentally enter and, in trust, sentiently seek nature's wisdom. You discover that your immediate natural attractions may differ from the attractions in your preconceived new-brain story. In addition, your attractions change to fulfill your inner nature's moods and yearnings moment by moment.

Spontaneously following and enjoying natural attractions enhances your new-brain's ability to trust sensory messages from the natural world via your inner nature. That trust encourages the new brain to validate these connections. Thank your natural senses for helping you reach green-in-green. Too often in today's stressful world we don't choose to responsibly make space for reconnecting and seeking natural attractions for their good feelings. They need our new-brain support to feel safe from wranglers.

For 15 minutes or more walk through this natural area by continuously following immediate natural attractions. Let the sentient callings of the next immediate attraction guide you. Immediately thank each calling for existing, guiding you, and giving you good feelings.

Some participant's reactions:

"This natural area feels like a web of interconnecting sensations right now. It feels really good."

"Life feels honest. The woodland feels like an extension of myself, like it's actually me."

"Thinking of plants and animals as relatives goes beyond metaphor. I genuinely feel related to them. It feels better than I can remember feeling about my stressful family at home."

"The realness of my natural attraction sensations makes it hard for me to believe that the rocks and trees aren't sensing something, too."

"I felt like I was a compass needle swinging towards the nameless attraction connections in the area, yet they responded to what I was. I was hot, so water's coolness attracted me."

"It feels like my life is a gently woven knot consisting of the sensory strands of nature."

"I see that connecting with nature takes place only in the moment and what I consciously or unconsciously need in that moment determines what attracts me and then fulfills me."

Write down the three most important things you learned from this activity.

Write three green-in-green statements that come from doing this activity.

How would you feel about having your ability to create and enjoy this feeling taken away?

What effect does this activity have on your sense of self-worth?

Chapter Eighteen

A Chapter of Your Life

In nature, our 53 natural senses know how to bring us to where we want to be.

Start this chapter by doing the following activity:

Activity 18: Sensing Like Nature

Go to an attractive natural area. Become involved with it and gain its consent to help you with this activity. If the area remains attractive, thank it.

Gently rub your hands across the top of your head and imagine that your hands are collecting your nature-separated, new-brain stories. Shake your hands in the air and discard these disconnected stories into the environment. Let its wisdom begin to recycle them. Repeat this procedure a few times and validate that with these stories gone, that you and nature are identical.

Now, with these stories gone, walk through this attractive natural area for 15 minutes. Have your new brain tell itself a new nature-centered story. This story says that as you walk through this natural area, you are walking through your own mentality and body. All of nature that you sense and feel around you is also inside you. It is often wrangled out of your awareness by society's expectations. In this natural area, you are walking into your subconscious. Note how attractions here feel and create nature-centered thinking.

In this natural area, any human-made objects or changes that may gain your attention on this walk are also attractions. They are the new-brain stories that, when the activity began, you discarded along with their effects on you. Note how they feel. Whether they feel comfortable or uncomfortable, thank each of them as you find them for what they teach you. Appreciate how they direct you in this moment.

Share your thoughts feelings and reactions to this activity in your journal and with companions. When possible, do this activity with a companion and share what you think and feel as you do it. Try not to distort your companion's observations or feelings. Ask for their permission to become involved with them, gain their consent to help you with this activity. Relate through your attractions to their inner nature, not to bad feelings from their external words or appearance.

Write down the three most important things you learned from this activity. Write three green in green statements that come from doing this activity. How would you feel about having your ability to create and enjoy this G/G taken away? What effect does this activity have on your sense of self-worth?

Now it is time for you to write this last chapter. In it, review and integrate the experiences you have had through this book. Think about what was important to you and the nature-connected statements that you have created. Blend them with your personal and professional life every day.

Appendices

Appendix A

Transitioning to Nature-Centered Thinking

A mother who felt the world was too violent kept her newborn child in a closet to protect her. When the child was discovered, at age 19, she had bonded to the closet. She was "in tune" with it and afraid to leave it. The child's self-identity, story, and beliefs might have been:

"I am a person that loves to sit on a closet shelf."
"I get good feelings from rubbing a doorknob."
"I like it in here...I can survive here."
"Outside is a violent, unsafe place."

Many of the child's normal senses for gaining satisfaction in society were withdrawn or missing. A few years after being removed from the closet, the child died, unable to adapt. Unfortunately, this metaphor parallels too many case histories.

Like being closeted, our excessively indoor lives teach us to relate to the natural world insensitively and inappropriately. We experience a constant flow of signals to this effect. They are green-in-orange tensions (G/O). Earth and our G/O tensions may recover from our closeting through green-in-green (G/G) experiences, stories, and relationships. They are based on sensing natural attractions in a natural area.

IMPORTANT: Caution should be taken to stay involved with natural attractions only. Be sensitive. If an attraction dissipates or becomes unattractive, immediately find and follow a new attraction.

The competency to enjoy positive relationships within and around us develops from reconnecting with nature and producing G/G statements. Well constructed G/G statements contain the elements needed to expose and educate our closeted new brain to natural values available outside. Psychologically and physically, G/G statements help move us out of our indoor thoughts and lives and the adverse relationships they tend to produce. One Reconnecting With Nature participant recently wrote:

> "Earlier in the course, I wrote that during my childhood I learned that my self in the moment was just what I couldn't trust - that my self was utterly not trustable - I would do or say something 'wrong' or I would hurt someone's feelings or be hurt or lose my temper and feel the pain, etc. I did feel this pain for years and years. Learning to trust my senses and attractions and validations of those connections with nature and myself in the moment is wonderful. I continue to expand the use of this process into every moment. It is perhaps the greatest gift I have received from this course. When I am green-in-green, I can be. When I am truly me I can trust me not to hurt or be hurt."

The elements of a strong green-in-green statement and areas it addresses are, at first, attainable by valuing and using the basic statement: My experience in nature shows me that I am a person who gets good feelings (from, when, by, etc.) _____. Its elements enable us to bring into consciousness the following closeted areas:

ELEMENT	CLOSETED AREA ADDRESSED
My	sense of self and connectedness
experience	multisensory, hands-on, trustable information in the moment
in nature	the natural world, not an indoor new brain story, is the source of this information
shows me	reasonable new-brain and old-brain experience, balance, and validation
I am	self identity
a person who gets	human identity, interactiveness, openness, connectedness, natural functioning

good feelings	sensory positive feedback within nature operating and responsive, trustable, worthwhile, connected to wholeness
from	ability to relate to nature in new brain and old brain balance

Society restrictively programs our screen of conscious awareness to think, relate, and know life through new brain reasoning and verbal language. The G/G statement above attempts to assimilate nature's wisdom into our new-brain thinking. The quicker we develop the ability to create a reliable G/G new brain story base that establishes our identity as citizens of Earth, the sooner we will be able to build and sustain G/G relationships with ourselves, society, and nature. As we build G/G experiences, we will also begin to share and teach it. That is a path to living responsibly. It is how natural people participate in the global life community in balance with other species.

I suggest that it is reasonable to use the basic G/G statement as a check point for developing the G/G statement habit: "My experience in nature shows me that I am a person who gets (generates, senses, discovers) good feelings (trust, nurturing, joy, belonging)."

Our great challenge is to recognize that the G/G feeling on the color chart is a metaphor. Real G/G only comes from nature itself, not substitutes like the chart's words and colors. G/G from substitutes often bond or addict us. They become a fix that is a product of disconnected stories, not nature's wisdom.

Once G/G is established, the challenge becomes: "What immediate actions can I take to sustain my relationships. How can I participate in these actions now?"

Examples of basic G/G statements: Caution: Do not measure yourself against the following statements. Each reconnecting with nature activity you do brings you to a space where you will naturally produce green-in-green statements that are right for you. Examples:

My experience in nature shows me that I am a person who gets good feelings:

from this flower and knowing that when I am in nature, my mind is peaceful and I am centered.

by holding this tree and being moved emotionally when I thank the tree for its presence and friendship.

by lying on this mossy rock in the sun and sensing that nature helps me to really feel.

as I watch a small area in nature and see how everything moves and flows. I am flowing with it as my natural self, being nature, being unconcerned about my appearance, being in a non-verbal, non-judgmental way and enjoying it.

Enriched G/G statements: To intensify and solidify the impact and value of a G/G statement, respond to the statement: "I would not be willing to give up my ability to experience this connection because _____." Ask yourself what it would mean to you or how you would feel if this G/G connection-sensation was taken away.

Summary: To produce powerful G/G statements:
1. Go to an attractive natural area, the more natural the better.
2. Gain permission from the area to relate to it.
3. Do the activity. Only make non-verbal contact with attractions.
4. Note the sensory fulfillment generated and express appreciation for these good feelings.
5. Write and share statements describing how the activity felt and makes sense to you.
6. Describe how you would feel to lose the ability to have these experiences.
7. Get at least one night of sleep before you do the next activity.

The following statements were written by a participant taking the e-mail Reconnecting With Nature course and summarize the value of creating G/G statements:

"Three important things that I learned from doing this activity are:

1) Nature created and gives us the ability to know and feel the difference between G/G and G/O so that we can detect when we are in or out of balance/harmony with nature.

2) Our problems are the result of our mentality's separation from our

attractive, supportive, natural origins and their inherent wisdom.

3) To make changes when we/society are off balance, we must discard old, irresponsible stories and honor the wisdom from the old brain's sensate connections with nature."

Notice that the following statements do not use the model sentence above, but cover the same ground.

1) In nature, I like feeling the power of validating my sensory experiences, as another form of connection to the oneness of all things. I would be saddened to lose this power because I would lose contact with an important part of myself.

2) I love the sensation of balance/harmony that comes to me when I listen to the wisdom and guidance of my connection to nature. It would hurt me to be deprived of it because it would rob me of contact with a balanced community that I respect.

3) I honor the power of my old brain and new brain to work together in providing me the opportunity to live in integrity. I would deeply feel the loss of being human if someone took this sense from me.

Islands of reason: Each statement helps bring your inner nature's intelligence and energy into your new brain consciousness where it is accessible to you. Once there, the senses of reason, language, and consciousness welcome and celebrate. That is why G/G always feels good. Good means "connected with the whole." G/G unites the long separated family of senses. Remember that reason, language, and consciousness are natural senses, too. Wranglers have herded them together and corralled them into the new brain story of conquering nature and the old brain.

G/G statements demand the new brain produce integrity. Imagine each statement to be a lifesaving flotation pillow supporting a life raft in the sea of consciousness. The more buoyant the life raft, the greater the size, support, and resiliency of the network of natural attraction relationships.

You can produce optimized statements by having it contain each of the 10 following components:

-create and write it from attractions in natural areas,
-have it identify yourself and other species,
-validate that it produces good feelings,
-name the natural senses involved,
-thank these natural senses,
-thank the natural areas and things involved,
-state how you would feel being deprived of this experience,
-read these statements aloud to yourself,
-share it with another person and seek reactions to it,
-get at least one night's sleep before you make more G/G statements.

Once you've developed a portfolio of statements, you find that the "life raft" improves your thinking, resiliency, and confidence. It and nature become your close friends.

A penny for your thoughts (and feelings):

Place a penny (okay, in this day and age it may de a dime!) in a jar for each lifesaver you place in your G/G "life raft." At 100 coins, take the money and spend it in a way that will help you involve others in the G/O to G/G process.

The G/O to G/G checklist and other additional growth tools:

You may further encourage your disconnected new brain thinking to include nature by responding to the following questions regarding a G/G experience or statement:

-Did you ask the natural area for permission to visit it? How do you know it gave permission? Did you thank it for its permission?

-How do you thank nature for having "invented" your old brain ability to feel?

-Why do you deserve to have and enjoy green-in-green experiences?

-Do you consciously identify and thank the specific natural senses involved in this G/G for being? (Chapter 5) For generating good feelings?

-How do you feel when you say your statement aloud?

-How do you feel sharing it with others?

-Who do you think might benefit if you shared your statements with them?

-If you feel relief from this experience, what is being relieved?

-What would you sense if this G/G experience was eliminated from your life?

-Do you invite other people to involve themselves in this kind of experience?

-Does this help you better know part of yourself you may have ignored? What part?

-Does your G/G statement contain phrases such as: I like, I love, I appreciate, I discover, I thank?

-Did this experience arise from contact with the inner nature of another person?

-Are you determining what immediate actions you can take to sustain your green-in-green relationships. Are you engaging in these actions?

Appendix B

A Case History of RWN

True recovery occurs when we acknowledge our multisensory self
and let nature nurture it.

The green-in-orange to green-in-green transition works as a preventative for disorders and a catalyst for enjoying responsible relationships. In this appendix, I share the use of the activities and G/O to G/G process in recovery work–the sad, extremely challenging setting of impoverished young people at risk with drug and alcohol related disorders. The number of such young people is rising. They are wounded battlefield victims of a society unofficially at war with nature, a war we seldom admit exists but whose effects speak for themselves. It is difficult for these youngsters to participate in relationships because stories activate wranglers within them and hurt them so easily. They are vulnerable.

The moment an individual chooses to enter a nature-centered relationship, they inherently begin to feel good. In that moment the story world disappears along with some of its stress. They have filled that moment's screen of consciousness with supportive attraction feelings, a natural sensory wisdom that is intelligent enough not to deny or attack itself. As these relationships continue, not only do they become a habitual way of thinking and relating, they also improve the health of the natural world so that the present war zone begins to become more peaceful. Although this sounds like it promotes an addictive dependency on the natural environment, the process works equally as well in reconnecting us with our own and other people's inner nature as it does in reconnecting with the environment. Our lives, health, and happiness are dependent on nature's life and health.

The following nature reconnecting article describes the work of Kurtland Davies, a high school counselor, and myself, in injecting the nature reconnecting process into a drug and alcohol program for students at risk:

A public school workshop: Monday, January 30, 1995, 11:15 A.M., Vancouver, Washington, U.S.A.

As if the wisdom of nature has us in mind, the rain clouds part and sunshine-washed blue sky lets the local park glow in its inherent beauty. In attendance here are a group of at-risk high school students along with their teachers, their counselor, and myself, a guest instructor.

Smoking cigarettes and hesitating to get too close to me or each other, the group gathers within hearing distance at my request. My challenge is to introduce some elements of reconnecting with nature to these students as well as demonstrate the value of the process and its remarkable effects. The significance of this demonstration is that this group, with the exception of its teachers, consists of victims of Western Culture's nature-separated dream; they are young people fed up with society's expectations. They are either chemically dependent, unwed mothers, violent, co-dependent, harboring food disorders, apathetic, or a combination of these troubles. Most have low self-esteem. All are traditional school dropouts now attending an alternative education program that sponsors this nature connecting hour in the park with me. Ironically, many parks are closed at night because of the threat from the presence of people at risk, people this group represents.

We gather together around a picnic table and I ask the students and staff to think about a conversation that recently occurred. I say:

Last week, a student named Bill told me that he was positive that nature was unfriendly, dangerous and "a bitch." Bill's feelings came from a camping trip this fall. He climbed up a cliff and felt scared of nature because if the rock crumbled or he made a false move, nature would injure or kill him. While he climbed the cliff, nature rained on him and he got wet and cold. Another day he was hiking without a shirt and it got so cold and windy that he nearly froze. He also walked balancing on rocks by a rushing creek when slime on one caused him to fall into the water and nearly be washed away. It reminded him of on the beach last summer when the waves almost carried him away. 'For sure, nature is no friend,' he said."

Smirking, but concerned, the students tell me Bill was either a freak or just trying to be cool. They ask if this "dude" was doing drugs, "Something is wrong with the dweeb because he put himself in dangerous situations, and rather than see what a jerk he is, he blamed his troubles on nature," they conclude. They summarize that Bill was a danger to himself, it was not nature's fault that all this bad stuff happened.

I say to these students and teachers: "The nature connecting activity we will do now asks you to avoid Bill's nonsense. What I want you to do is be sensible in nature. Look around this natural area and find a place that attracts you because it feels like you'll enjoy it and because it is safe. By yourself, explore it for ten minutes. Try to really know it many ways, through many senses: touch, taste, smell and sight. Then we'll get together and share what happens during this short solo."

In ten minutes, the group returns. Changes in them are immediately apparent. Most are at ease, smiling and not shy about getting close so they can hear each other. "Is anybody missing?" I ask. They look around and even though they had never been together as a group before, they somehow know that Charley and Sarah are not there. As we do a head count, from different directions first Charley then Sarah come into view.

"Can you tell each other how you feel and what you think right now?" I ask the group. They respond in as follows:

I feel really peaceful, this little park is peaceful.
I feel part of something.
I had a good time.
It was so beautiful.
I trust that tranquil place and nature.
I felt parts of myself that have been missing since I was younger.
I feel happy right now.
I like being here now with the group more.
Right now I feel like I'm being, simply truly being.
I think we shouldn't smoke while going into nature.
I picked up some garbage, it was a downer seeing it.
I feel more alive and like living.
I feel centered.
We should do this activity further from the city, from the noise and houses nearby.
I wish I could live like this all the time.
I'd like to get a job where I work outside in nature and help protect it.
I feel gentle right now, yet I was uncool when we first got here.
I feel like doing things that wouldn't hurt this place, that would respect it.
It would be less expensive to live close to nature. I'd be willing to risk it.
I feel pure and clean even though I've been sitting in dirt.
I sense a certain spirit here that I don't feel elsewhere.
I sense that how we think and feel right now is a fact as real and true as $2 + 2 = 4$.

The teacher who leads the grief group at school notices that a pine tree has been planted in the park as a memorial to someone. It stands by itself in the middle of a lawn near a plaque. This attracts and saddens her. "I think the pine must be lonely," she says. "It's not in a forest of trees, in a community."

I ask the group: "If you were that pine tree, what might you be experiencing at this moment?" Here is what they say:

I'd like the joy and warmth of the sunlight.

I'd have the fun of the wind blowing through me.

I'd feel close to the soil, supported, rooted, grounded.

I wouldn't feel competitive because I'd be so far away from the roots of trees in the forest.

I'd be happy that I lived in a protected park area, I wouldn't worry about being hurt or cut down.

I'd enjoy the sound of birds singing and children laughing here in the park.

I would be proud that somebody noticed me and cared about me and thought of me as memory to somebody they loved.

I'd dance in the beauty of all the sparkling drops of water on my limbs.

I think I would be happy because I'm not in the shadow of all the large forest trees. I'm a pine tree and I usually can't grow in the shade of other trees.

The group does not support the teacher's grief story, rather the experience in nature lets them independently create and validate their own story. This is the same group of young people who ordinarily make the park and our streets hazardous places. From this hour in nature, these same young folks feel attracted to nature and to each other for we have found something responsible, something basic we hold in common. We affirm that we trust our moments connected to natural attractions in the environment and each other.

Adult or student, the group looks forward to continuing this nature connecting activity class during the coming school year. They say they want to learn additional activities and ways of thinking that would let Earth teach them how to intensify and preserve the good way they think and feel in this moment.

Discussion

Not by accident, the right touch of nature works a magic that may be used as a preventative. Throughout the year, participants of all ages respond as these students did to Project NatureConnect e-mail or correspondence courses . Using a self-guiding training manual, each participant does one of 109 nature-connecting activities. Then they validate their thoughts and feelings by sharing it with six other people on the course, some of whom may live in different countries. Participants complete the activity by sharing with each other what they think and feel about the contact they have with each other. They end up gaining support from nature and each other and they learn to teach the process to others as well.

From the standpoint of mental health, G/O to G/G acts as a self-abuse and social-abuse preventative. With these students at risk, we use it as a cure for chemical abuse. Counselor Kurtland Davies describes the process in the following paragraphs from his article about the program:

"In the spring of 1995, a group of eight poverty level drug affected high school 'at risk' students participated in an experimental 10 week nature-centered multisensory counseling program. Its purpose was twofold: First to disconnect participants from dependency on drugs and alcohol; second to reconnect participants' inner nature with the natural environment to rejuvenate their natural wisdom and resiliency.

One day, during a tag game, Sara was hit in the face with a nerf ball. She was not hurt, but immediately started screaming at John, who had thrown the ball. John yelled back and Sally took his side, joining in the noise. Jim and Alisha stood and stared, frozen. Kurtland, the counselor, yelled "STOP!," and gathered all of them into a circle.

What unfolded was a series of "G/O stories" that had taken each student out of the moment and into the past without them being aware of it. Immediately before the incident, they were enjoying the interactive flow of their natural senses of fun, community, power, movement and balance, to name only a few. Then an innocent event disintegrated that flow in one second.

Kurtland asked Sara what feelings she was experiencing. She recognized anger, fear, frustration, humiliation. He asked her if these feelings were familiar. She quickly realized that she was reliving feelings she had as a child when she was hit in the face by an abusive family member. This and similar situations created one of her stories, which is: "Something is wrong with me. I don't fit in. I will be punished (G/O)." She reacted, not to the present situation, but to the old story, triggering other G/O stories in her friends.

When John became the target of Sara's attack, he went into his own story. When he experienced abuse as a child, he learned to survive by fighting back, arguing, and provoking conflict: "I'll get hurt if I don't defend myself. No one will help me." Sally soon became aware that she was playing out her story of rescuing and codependency: "If I take care of him, he'll take care of me." Jim and Alisha began to understand that when strong negative emotions are expressed, their stories tell them: "The safest thing to do is to hide." Jim felt powerless in the face of beatings by his stepfather and Alisha learned early to make herself small and fade into the background in order to survive in an alcoholic family system.

As the group members shared the feelings that were stimulated by their old memories, they saw how we all carry unresolved G/O "life stories" that have pain attached to them. They learned how we hide these stories in our subconscious to avoid feeling their pain when we become conscious of them. When a situation reminds us of a similar past one, our subconscious mind tries to protect us. It brings onto our screen of consciousness similar past stories and senses to warn us of possible danger, to tell us to seek other natural attractions. This reaction is as fixed and automatic as smelling a lemon making us salivate. Even when we are involved in a supportive situation, unexpected stress triggers similar protective stress stories. Painful stories appear on our screen of consciousness and we relive the unresolved pain attached to these memories until we change the old stories, or move into new stories that assure us of the safety available in the present moment.

Framework

This nerf ball incident occurred during a project designed for "students at risk." The goal was to disconnect participants from drug use and reconnect them to the natural world, their own true nature, and their natural sense of community. The theoretical framework was taken from Dr. Michael Cohen's Applied Ecopsychology model which suggests that intimate old brain contact with nature puts people immediately in touch with an innate wisdom that when validated by the new brain affects a deep healing of self.

The ecological web of life is based on consensus. The word means "a general agreement," and it comes from Latin words meaning "to feel with." In consensus, every being in the system consents, on a sensory level, to participate fully in the process of cooperative community survival and growth through their natural senses. Without a verbal story to guide them, each individual's survival depends upon the energizing sensory and metabolic support available to them in any given moment. The individuals who sustain the greatest cooperative support relationships with their surroundings survive. Adverse aspects of their environment are, at some level, attracted to transform into support for them. They drift out of a sense of survival of self and into a sense of survival of all. In congress, these attraction sensitivities move to ensure the survival of all populations, predator and prey alike. Through continual multisensory interactions, all sense that they are part of a larger organism, Earth's ecosystem.

The students in this program were "Indoor Sapiens," meaning that they were cut off from the natural world and the many sensory attractions that could nurture and balance them. Reared in this atmosphere of stress and internal war, the students create and live in their G/O stories of survival which remove them from enjoying their cooperative multisensory lives.

Activities

The students experienced many of Dr. Cohen's activities. As their old and new brain communicated, their stress seemed to melt away. They particularly enjoyed the guided nature walk activity. One student closed their eyes, eliminating dependency on the sense of sight, while another acted as "nature guide." Neither could speak, which prevented new brain communication, so the guide had to direct by touch only. The guides led their partners into the world of smell, touch, taste, moisture, and many other senses of nature. If the guides wanted their partners to see something, they squeezed their shoulder. The "blind" partner opened their eyes for only a second and then shut them. After ten minutes, the students switched roles. The numerous natural sensations that this activity awakened began to bond the partners to each other and to nature. They rediscovered their many hidden natural senses.

Because we learn to think in language, it was important to talk about each activity afterward. The new brain validated the sensory attractions of the old brain, which added greatly to each experience. From this process, old abuse stories were exposed and the seeds of new stories were planted in the enjoyment of nature-connected moments. In one activity, the students went into a natural area to find a specific attraction such as a brook, tree, flower, or stone. When they found the attraction, they completed the following sentence: "I like _____ (the attraction) because _____." As they shared their sentences with each other, they were reminded that they, too, are nature. They were asked to repeat the sentence, changing it to say: "I like myself because _____," using the same list of attributes. At first they resisted, not believing their own words, but they soon began to see the truth in their statements since they were nature, too. Each statement they made about themselves felt good.

In the above activity, Eileen was attracted to a delicate wildflower "because it is beautiful and perfect." When she said, "I like myself because I am beautiful and perfect," she quickly added, "and no one tells the flower that it's ugly and a drug addict." Nature was telling her that she was beautiful and perfect, but her old story was telling her she was ugly and defective. As she talked about this old story and allowed herself to feel the hurt it had caused her, a space was made for a new healthy story to grow within her. She became more aware of and supported by the natural environment.

Often, the stories of "students at risk" block their natural senses of trust, power, community, nurturing, self, grief, and pain, among others. This triggers the natural empathy, community, and nurturing attractions of the staff to enable these students to responsibly participate in our local community. We developed a program specifically designed to work with and recover their natural senses.

The design of Project Reconnect incorporated three phases. Phase One involved three weeks of play. There was no pressure to do; rather, only encouragement to be to be creative and playful. In this safe and supportive environment, many story-blocked natural senses were unleashed and rejuvenated. Stronger senses of trust and community began to develop. Also, a sense of grief was opened up as the students felt the pain of abusive childhood experiences and the loss of the childhood fulfillment of their many natural attractions. Our challenge was to get the students into the present moment where they could rejoice because they could now choose to feel these multisensory attractions and then actually fulfill them.

Phase Two helped students to reconnect to their old brain ways of knowing, to begin to make peace with them and integrate them with their new brain indoor stories. Dr. Cohen's activities were formally introduced during this phase and continued to be used throughout the rest of the program.

Phase Three consisted of five days on a challenge course (known as the "Ropes Course"), where the students learned team work, problem solving, and how to release stress and fear to find power and joy. In this phase, one of the biggest challenges for the group was the five foot trust fall. Not many groups take on this initiative because of its high challenge to each individual's hurt senses of trust and its requirement for a well focused, efficient and trustworthy team. The task is as follows. Each person climbs up a five foot platform, turns and faces away from the group. Then, on a signal, they fall backwards into the arms of their teammates. This was a particularly productive initiative. Each student was taken out of the support in the moment by their new brain story which produced fear by telling them they would be injured. Automatically, stories of past betrayals flooded their consciousness. They spoke their fears out loud. Their teammates responded to their own natural attractions to nurture and support them by allowing them to feel their emotions fully and reassuring them. They also spoke these out loud, calling out the names of natural senses they were feeling. Each student was eventually able to get back into the immediate moment of natural attraction to their senses of safety, trust, and belonging and fell into the support of their community. Everyone's natural senses gave consent to cooperatively fulfill themselves by and through everyone involved in the community. Afterwards, each participant, including the instructors, felt a sense of exhilaration and personal power.

On the last day of the ropes course, each student consented to complete certain activities on the "high elements," based on their own level of personal challenge. Some walked poles and wires suspended 25 to 30 feet in the air. Some jumped off the top of a 25 foot pole onto a trapeze. During these activities, fears were induced by stories that block fulfillment of many senses, such as distance, place, gravity, community, and trust. Their new brain was attracted to reason in order to guide them safely. It created new stories to make sense of the situation by relying on their restored old brain natural senses of community, trust, belonging, consciousness, balance, physical ability, and self as well as those of their reconnect group.

The final phase of the project was a three day wilderness outing. Because of unexpected weather and terrain, the outing became a huge challenge. Each student was forced to look inward to find natural attractions for survival, strengths they did not know they had. They functioned like a healthy ecosystem. When one student got into trouble, another student was eager to help them through the crisis. They carried each others' packs, encouraged each other when tired, and gave each other a hand over steep parts of the trail. Every student later said that they did not want to let the group down. Their natural attractions to being in nature, community, and nurturing the group pushed them onward when they wanted to quit. They felt closer as a group and stronger as individuals.

Further Discussion

Many outdoor education models teach students to manage stress by pushing through it, conquering it. For example, if you have a fear of heights, you face the fear by walking a cable high in the air. If you fear abandonment and injury, you dare to fall backwards into the arms of your teammates to establish trust. These are stressful experiences which can help build teamwork, trust, community, and self-esteem. However, if these experiences are not put into the proper context or do not include sufficient emotional support, they encourage the "Conquer Your Fear" story.

When the students experienced severe weather conditions and tough terrain on the trip and had to keep going, it could have reinforced their idea that nature is dangerous and hard and it is necessary to push through and conquer it. It could have reinforced the dominant cultural stories of "just do it," "no pain/no gain," "winner takes all," "nice guys finish last," "don't cry out loud," etc. We create pain, fear, and stress from our old cultural and family stories that push through our natural bonds, that separate us from our true nature rather than respecting it. This tends to perpetuate our painful separation from nature and our continued abuse of the environment and each other. This is why we added the energy of Dr. Cohen's Applied Ecopsychology. Without this nature-centered psychological element, outdoor education has the potential to add to our problems rather than ameliorate them.

Dr. Cohen's ecopsychology story is not to conquer nature, but to flow, dance, and balance with nature and each other. Nature consists of attractions. Pain, fear, and stress are natural attractions, part of nature's perfection. These natural discomforts are nature's way of telling us we don't have sensory support in this moment. They attract us to follow other immediate natural attachments. On the trip, our discomforts in nature intensified our natural attractions to nurturing, community, and trust. They supported our survival.

Findings

The results of the program were overwhelmingly positive. The students' growth was later reflected in the improved psychological test scores and analysis which show lower depression and drug use and higher self-esteem. Tests included the Beck Depression, Stress Test, Coopersmith Self-Esteem, Barksdale Self-Esteem, Sleep Inventory. The students now personally own activities and rationale for reconnecting with each other and with nature in the environment. Their challenge, and ours as instructors, is to continue to support each other and the environment as part of our daily lives.

The state of Earth and its people indicates that mentally and environmentally, we are distressed. These results suggest that nature-reconnecting activities used in daily stress situations could serve as an ecologically sound citizenship education program, a preventative for chemical, food, social and environmental abuse.

Analysis of Pre and Post Data

Student #1 has shown a most impressive improvement in all areas. This was the student who struggled the most on the high elements of the challenge course and had the most difficulty hiking up the mountain during the wilderness trip.

Student #2 has also shown steady improvement in all areas. In particular, she made progress on the Depression Inventory even though she was unable to participate in the final hike due to family obligations.

Student #3 has shown progress or stayed the same in each score. The Depression Inventory scores indicate more empowerment. This student showed a remarkable athletic ability and was extremely important to the group, especially on the challenge course. Although he showed no improvement in scores on the Self-Esteem test, there was one significant change. On the pre-test, he indicated that there were a lot of things about himself that he would change if he could, whereas on the post-test he indicated that this was no longer true.

Student #4 shows significant improvement on all scales. This student, like student #1, had to go through a lot of fear on the ropes course and hiking down the wilderness trail.

Student #5 missed taking a pre-test on stress. Those tests that were completed show improvement across the board. This student came into the program with a pretty healthy self-esteem. One reason is that he is the only student with a fairly stable home life.

Student #6 has shown improvement in all areas except for the sleep inventory. This student is in foster care and has some mixed feelings about returning to live with her mother. She was the youngest of our group and gained a lot of confidence. However, her anxiety about her family situation continues to show up in her sleep patterns.

In addition to the improved test scores, every students' attendance and academic progress improved while they were in Project Reconnect. No indications of chemical abuse were observed 60 days after the program ended.

Student Comments

"The program has shown me a way to stay clean through supportive friends and alternative activities such as the ropes course, hiking, etc.... basically getting in touch with nature and having a sense of team work, knowing someone is always going to be there for me."

"I learned that there is more in life than drugs. And that life can still be good (better) without them. It also boosted my self-esteem and showed me it's okay to be me. I hope that this will be an option for others next year."

"We did many things that have helped me learn about

myself. It has helped me overcome some great fears of mine. I used to be really insecure. Now I feel, and know, I can do anything I set my mind to. It has also helped me learn how to work as a group and be comfortable expressing my feelings. It was a great chance for me to become in touch with myself."

"It has helped me greatly in the past few months. It has kept me sane when I thought I wasn't and the group also reintroduced me to someone I haven't known in a long time: myself. A few of the most meaningful parts of this program were Project Adventure (ropes course), the hikes and the wilderness trip. Project Adventure showed me I could do things I never thought of being possible. And the hikes taught me many important skills to survive in the wild. I also learned to appreciate myself as a part of nature. So, in closing, I really owe a lot to this program for what it taught me about myself, my friends, and nature."

Epilogue

During Dr. Cohen's Project NatureConnect workshop with one of our recovery groups, we visited a damaged natural area next to the student's proposed new school. The area where we did the nature-reconnecting permission activity was slated to be paved as a parking lot (activity 2). As a result, the student's felt that the area, like themselves, wanted to recover from the abuse it had received from society. They sensed that it had been, in their words: "hurt, molested, invaded and trespassed," "it wanted to become healthy or die," "it felt trashed and overwhelmed," "it had no power, it needed help to recover." Since then, the area and their inner nature has given them permission to enlist the support of social and environmental agencies to save the area from becoming a parking lot. Instead the garbage will be removed and it will recover as an indigenous natural area. It will be nurtured and nurturing, support wildlife, an educational and therapeutic nature sanctuary for the school, and a host for doing these sensory nature reconnecting activities.

The students recently wrote and received a grant to help make this dream of theirs a reality. Here's what they said in the grant's vision statement:

"We are a recovery group based on reconnecting with nature. In our recovery efforts, nature plays a major role. We have chosen a small piece of wilderness that reflects us as a community. This wild community is being choked by alien plants and stressed by pollution, abandonment, and major loss. We, too, are being choked by drugs and stories that pollute our natural self. We feel abandoned by our society and cut off from nature which fills us with grief. As we remove the garbage, thorns, and ivy we will work on removing the toxins from our lives. As we plant healthy trees, we will learn new healthy ways to survive. By protecting this ecosystem we will find the strength to open our minds, hearts, and souls for the survival of our Mother Earth and ourselves."

The reader may not be as hurt and vulnerable as were the young people in this study. However, your challenge is the same as theirs on your own level. The challenge is to gain consent from your new brain to participate in the activities, to gain consent from nature in others and the environment to participate in life. Gaining consent to live can be seen as what every organism does to survive, no matter what its species.

Consider the G/O to G/G experiences these students had and their effects. Think about what our world would be like if 600 million people in it had RWN experiences with nature and their community, experiences that were similar to those enjoyed by these students. That thought is the essence of the RWN factor and it is shared by every member of the global life community. The sense in that thought is the love of life, an essence of the students, their classmates, and their teachers.

Acknowledgments

Project Reconnect was a joint program of Pan Terra Alternative High School, Vancouver, Washington and the Clark County Drug and Alcohol Center. The participants were drug or alcohol affected students that met for six hours a week in a drug and alcohol program at CDAC. This component of the Project, led by Ruth Queirolo and Cookie Quink, greatly contributed to its success. The ropes phase was guided by Project Adventure, Inc. staff members. Michael J. Cohen, Ed.D. Director, Project NatureConnect, acted as consultant and with Gaia Davies edited the manuscript. Catherine Freer Wilderness Therapy Expeditions provided excellent outdoor specialists who contributed to the survival and growth of the students and school counselor. The project utilized state funds provided through EPSDT and was administered through the Clark County Department of Community Services Alcohol and Drug Program. Kurtland Davies, School Counselor, Pan Terra HS, developed the play therapy. He also led the Project NatureConnect activities, the ropes course, and the wilderness outing. For further information, contact Kurtland Davies via Project NatureConnect.

Appendix C

An Ecology of Spirit

The reconnecting with nature process is a new brain story that says "It is reasonable to participate in the process of tapping into nature's balanced intelligence. It is reasonable to learn to think with that intelligence since it evokes comfortable feelings and has the wisdom avoid our runaway problems."

Nature-reconnected thinking allows our natural senses to produce a database of culturally unadulterated stories based on trustable personal experiences with nature. Our challenge is to learn to think with sensory attraction stories that keep us connected to nature's Nameless-Intelligent-Attraction-Love (NIAL). If we do not do this, nature disconnecting words, images, and reasoning continue to capture and contaminate our thinking. They draw us into disconnected conceptual schemes and belief systems. For example, if we call a forest "board feet," that term attaches our thinking to something entirely different than if we call that same forest a cathedral.

Our words are from the new brain. They carry new brain values. Attach a name to the nameless and you consciously know it and relate to it as a name. Do you really know who you are without knowing yourself by your name? How many people know you namelessly?

Although all people hold NIAL in common, millions of people have died in wars and crusades. Their global neighbors have killed them because they attached different names and values to the nameless. Each of us has experienced this attachment phenomenon. Aren't you attached to your name, to your God? How hurt are we when somebody defames us even though they have not physically abused us? Our hurt demonstrates the power of sensory attachment bonds to stories. Until these bonds are released, nothing changes.

Industrial society's nature estranged stories preoccupy our screen of consciousness. They conflict with each other, create stress, and separate us from the NIAL that cements the global community together.

We are dependent on words, yet they never accurately convey the essence of the natural world. Its integrity is nameless. With respect to NIAL, words can not substitute for experiencing the real thing. Without being aware of it, I discovered the same basic truth by extensively living in nature as did Lao-tzu in 500 BC. He said "The name that can be named is not the eternal name. The nameless is the origin of Heaven and Earth."

Many people say that nature-reconnecting activities are a spiritual experience. They enhance spirituality. When they discuss them as such, spiritual story conflicts often arise. A vast majority of us are steeped in spiritual stories that validate our nature exploitative ways. These stories say it is humanity's duty to subdue the Earth, to dominate nature. They say this is the word of God. These stories validate our nature-conquering course, for each of us are of our God and blessed by our God .

For those of us who have learned to experience NIAL as a form of spirit, this chapter presents some stories to consider. I include them here to help our new brain think about spirituality from a G/O to G/G point of view. I do this with trepidation about discussing "God things." For some, they are not discussable. They are sensory attachments that reason alone can not change. If this chapter's stories help bring the reader into further enjoyment and benefits from participation in the G/O to G/G process, then it serves its purpose.

Psychology closely relates to spirit. The word psyche means air, spirit, or soul. Psychology means the study or logic of the emotions/spirit/soul. Ecopsychology extends the human soul to include its ties with the environment.

Our nature-conquering spiritual stories often emanate from sections of the Bible that our anti-nature bias emphasizes. Our leaders carefully selected the stories that would be allowed to become part of the Bible. It is an edited work that excludes many points of view that challenged our leader's anti nature bias. We seek our Bible's nature-disconnected stories. They provide spiritual support for our disconnectedness. They help us feel comfortable about how and why we inflict injuries upon nature in people and places, injuries that otherwise seem immoral or unethical.

There are spiritual scriptures and stories that affirm our nature connectedness. If you seek a spiritual journey that does not lead to today's conflicts and irresponsibility, you may find the following stories I discovered or deduced, to prove helpful:

Genesis states:

"....In the beginning God created the Heaven and the Earth.
....And the spirit of God moved upon the face of the waters.
....And the earth brought forth grass and herb yielding seed after his kind, and the tree yielding fruit whose seed was in itself.
.....And God created great whales and every living creature that moveth...and every winged fowl...And God blessed them saying, 'Be fruitful and multiply.'
.....And God made the beast of the earth...and every thing that crept upon the Earth.
.....And God saw that it was good."

According to this account, these were the first five days of creation in which the Creator manifests Earth. But the scriptures say that on the sixth day, before people are created, God speaks with somebody or some things present on that day. That's different than what the Creator did the first five days when the Creator acted alone. God refers to "us" and "our" in Genesis 1:26 on that sixth day as follows:

".....And God said 'Let us make man in our image, after our likeness.'"

Who or what is this "us" to whom God speaks? Since people have not yet been created, God can not be speaking to humanity. If we trust God's words in the scriptures, then we know that all that exists on that sixth day is God and God's creation. For this reason, God may be speaking to "Earth and everything that creepeth upon the earth," to the living natural kingdom and spirit God just created. When God speaks to us, God speaks to the natural world, to natural life as we know it. Researchers validate this conclusion. Some have discovered that the Bible's "us" comes from ancient Pantheist biblical scriptures that involve multiple nature gods.

In support of this biblical account, scientific reasoning offers some compelling evidence about "us" as the natural world. The evidence asks us to consider the possibility that in Genesis 1:26 the story says that life, the land, you and I, are Us, a collection of united non-languaged functions and parts of what we term "God." On this point, Biology, Paleontology, Geology, Physics, Anthropology, and Philosophy as well as many cultures and religions converge. They agree upon the general sequence of events conveyed in Genesis. They recognize that the human species did not create, but rather arose during or after the natural world was already established. This diverse multitude of inquiry suggests that we are a product of, a likeness of Us; we, the natural world, and God, are one, having "one Breath." (Ecclesiastes 3-19). Western civilization's God making human beings out of dust from the soil (Genesis 2:7) further confirms this. The word "human" has its roots in humus, a fertile forest soil. We and nature are Us, we innately know and love Us because we sense Us in each other through multiple nameless loves. Too often we forget that an infant knows NIAL at birth and before.

Converging evidence suggests that the Genesis sequence and its statement ".....And God said 'Let us make man in our image, after our likeness,'" spiritually and scientifically makes each of us a seamless continuum of the natural world. We and it are Us and Us has no name, no verbal language. Us is "The One that has no name" and the Bible sometimes identifies God that way in scriptures. Us, NIAL, and the nameless are synonymous. I use them interchangeably in this chapter. I do not however, capitalize the nameless for the same reason that we do not capitalize love or the wind, hills, or stars.

Nature reconnections help us experience that people and the nameless are created and sustained by the sensory wisdom we hold in common We learn not to see natural areas as different than people. The only difference is that people know, understand, and often relate through new brain language stories, a process foreign to NIAL. Individuals whose stories and lives validate NIAL neither sustain, suffer from, nor create many of the problems of those who live in separation from nature.

The Law of the Nameless

"The beginning of wisdom is calling things by their right name," said Confucius. In living outdoors and using sensory nature-connecting activities for thirty years, I have discovered a Law of the Nameless. The Law gives the right name to our Us-estranged lives. Apply it to places or people, and things change for the better. The Law incorporates and respects the wholeness of the nameless and every aspect of billion of years of our creative, evolving life process and spirit which we and Earth manifest.

Uniquely, The Law of the Nameless holds true for all members of the plant, animal, and mineral kingdoms. It states:

At any given moment:

-Everything desires to be.

-Natural attractions interconnect everything.

-Natural attraction relationships build stability.

The Law of the Nameless Part 1

Everything desires to be. Translation: everything is a being and consists of attraction relationships. According to modern physics, in the beginning of this universe, an annihilating struggle (the Big Bang?) took place between matter (material existence) and anti-matter. The nameless desire to be of "a small amount of matter won its fight to be as matter. That small amount of matter is all the matter that makes up our material universe," noted Albert Einstein and Noble Prize laureate George Wald. The vast majority of the universe is non-material attraction relationships. They are natural loves and marriages, manifesting themselves so strongly that they become solids, they materialize. The difference between the material and non-material is like the difference between trying to poke a pencil between your fingers when you hold your hand is still, versus when you very quickly vibrate your hand back and forth like a windshield wiper. The material world as we know it, including people, is made up of vibrant attraction relationships. It expresses and is an ongoing nameless desire to be itself, to be its process of being. People know the desire to be as a feeling or feelings of survival.

We need only attempt to change any aspect of Us, including ourselves, to discover the existence of stabilizing attraction forces that, in congress, intelligently, organize, preserve, and regenerate Us. We feel them. The only way we know anything is material is that we sense it to be material through touch, temperature, moisture etc. Things that register on our screen of consciousness through certain sensations, for example water, we call material. Things that register through other sensations, like language or thirst, we consider to be non-material. What all these things have in common is that they all register in consciousness as various sensations. Our story then labels them and places certain values on them.

Scientifically describing the physical world as an expression of a desire to be makes the physical universe a drive, a sense, a verb, an immediate motivated action that we feel. It is part of our soul for we are of it. Survival becomes not just accidental, random chance, mechanical or physical forces; rather, existence and growth at every level have a direction, meaning, and purpose. The purpose is to be attain higher diversity and thereby more stability and security. This nameless desire to be is our universe's underlying energy.

Often when it comes to understanding such speculative matters we say, "Only God knows, it's a God thing." Interestingly, in 1700 BC, as nature-gods and idols became taboo, our civilization's original One-God was called YHWH (Yahweh) which means The One Who Is. Language experts say the sound YHWH identifies "the non-languaged one," "the one who has no name." The word YHWH is a form of the ancient Sanskrit verb "to be." Yahweh not only was, or expressed the original desire to be, Yahweh may also be the source of the exclamation "Yahoo!" We consider God to be the essence of life and the word essence can mean "to be more fully."

In support of Yahweh being the desire to be, the early Bible says in Exodus 3-14 that Moses asked God /Yahweh to identify him or herself, and God said to Moses, "I AM THAT I AM...Tell the children of Israel 'I AM' sent you to them." I am is the verb "to be." Many spiritual people say, "God is being itself, to let ourselves be is to enter into union with God." You see, it is not simply by chance that we call ourselves human beings. And, as is demonstrated by the global life community seldom using language, natural being is mostly a non-language attraction experience that for people is sentient. We feel it.

The Law of The Nameless Part 2

Natural attractions hold everything together. Translation: every being is naturally attracted to continually form supportive relationships with its surroundings. In reality, all things, including materials, are actually beings in attraction relationships. Every being consists of a multiplicity of natural attraction relationships. Each thing is a relationship network that exists in the present moment. Each being sustains itself and/or grows through attractions, through "mutual consent marriages" into more complex and diverse relationships in order to exist with more stability. This natural attraction process sustains mineral compounds as well as organic and non material relationships. As matter establishes additional stabilizing attraction relationships, Us harmoniously becomes more secure, diverse, complex, and attractive.

Since its birth billions of years ago, the original universe has continually diversified. Its attractions have fused into amalgamations we call subatomic particles, atoms, elements, molecules, atmosphere, oceans, trees, mountains, species, people, weather systems, etc. All things are beings consisting mostly of atomic space filled with attraction energies. For example, some physicists claim that if you squeezed the attraction energy forces out of a mountain range, you would reduce the entire range to the size of a neutron. Each "thing" consists largely of attractions and is sensitive to new attractions. Each thing grows, diversifies, vibrates, and guides the universe in the moment.

The Law of The Nameless Part 3

Natural attraction relationships build stability. Translation: Every being, including any mineral, is always attracted directly, or by attraction chains, to every other being. The greater the number and diversity of mutually supportive attraction relationships a being has, the more stable and secure is its being, and the greater is its ability to cope with stresses. Without having some form of attractive connections, beings can't consent to grow or relate to each other. What we call natural repulsions, or negatives, guide us to natural attractions, to more stable, supportive, Us relationships. Our alienated stories about Us prevent us from recognizing this anti-entropy process.

A substantiation of the law of the nameless is that on a macro level, the natural world thrives without producing garbage, war, or insanity. This is no accident. Rather, it's because everything grows from loves, from everything's attractions to everything else. Everything is naturally attractive including each of us. This explains why, in the world of Us, nothing is rejected, unwanted, negative, unattractive, or unnecessary. There's no such thing as garbage, pollution, or excessive stress. Obviously, Us is a form of unconditional love in action.

Another substantiation of the law of the nameless is that when you make a value judgment about Us and remove what appears to be a detrimental part of Us, for example, a "predator," the total community deteriorates rather than improves. Again, this suggests that everything is attractive, wanted, and needed.

Obeying the Law of the Nameless

Let us now apply the law of the nameless to people. Every person is naturally that part of the universal desire to be which, through natural attractions, has over the eons evolved and materialized itself as a person. We each naturally personify the desire to be. We are each naturally attractive because we consist totally of attraction forces. However, our dependence upon surviving through disconnective stories that try to predict and control Us creates mechanistic, new-brain Newtonian words, logic, and reasoning. Through them we perceive the unconditional love process of Us as chaos because the nameless unpredictably adapts its totality to include every newly formed attraction relationship and change. In contrast, our sentient old-brain inner nature senses and celebrates the life-giving process of Us. It demands NIAL fulfillment. Our inner nature reasons through feelingful desires for "Yahoos," through attractive sensory "psycho-logic" relationships. Us in us seeks to enjoy the good feelings, wisdom, and power of nature's love. However, most of our tropicmaking indoor stories and reasoning disengage us from feelingly connecting to Us.

The stress from this conflict generates our most urgent problems.

In summary, our desire to be is a trustable, nameless, natural love we sometimes call survival. We each fulfill it by forming unique stabilizing, supportive relationships through our natural attractions to other beings. Every natural attraction helps support, stabilize, and secure our being. Good feelings signal that we are on that path. That's why satisfying our natural attractions feels good to us and why we deserve to have good feelings. Good diverse natural feelings, working in congress, are Us showing us our personal trail to survival in balance. This attractive sensory relationship and growth process, on some level, is the same process used by every other species. We only interrupt the process when we create, believe, or act out stories that don't respect it and disconnect us from Us.

Updating Creation

For the many people who, at least in part, experience the natural world spiritually, the law of the nameless suggests an updated creation story. The story reconciles spirit, science, and psychology. Because it supports multisensory holism, it neither assaults, exploits, nor engineers us or anything else. It says:

Billions of years ago, Yahweh, the nameless, attractive love To Be, desired a universe. Because Yahweh the cohesive Creation Force desired it to be, it materialized. That's how and why it is. Being of, by, and from an attractive God, an all-knowing Higher Power, our universe wisely and attractively creates and stabilizes through natural attractions. The very nature and attractiveness of the Great Circle of Life is both the Great Spirit's wisdom and His/Her unconditional love for this universe to be.

Noble laureate George Wald notes that Mind has always existed as a source and condition of physical reality. Every day, eclectic caring minds gather evidence which converges to confirm this creation story. For example, physicists now demonstrate that several basic attraction forces are unified into a single force (Yahweh?) when placed in environments that simulate the conditions of billions of years ago. Researcher's find that most of the material world actually consists of vibrating attraction energies which hold matter together. Some suggest that all the material matter that makes up this universe could be put into a space smaller than a volleyball, that what we call materials are actually strong solidified attraction marriages. The material world we so idolize, including ourselves, consists of throbbing attractions to be. To our cost, our culture's "conquer nature" survival stories seldom recognize or validate our natural attractions, the sensory substance of Us. When our stories, labels, or "conquer nature" logic block us from feelingful contact with Us, our troubles increase.

Nature reconnecting activities safely connect us with what some call spirit by validating Us, our innate attractions to nature that we feel but which defy description. We know nature as an act of God and "By His work the Master is known." Our great spiritual leaders spent much time in the wilderness. They met God there, not downtown. We celebrate their birth, deeds, and death. We now need to honor their extended periods of 40 days or more in the wilderness. Any person who seeks and spends 40 days alone in the wilderness will experience profound change for the better.

Connecting With The Nameless:

Nature-reconnecting techniques enable anyone to purposely reconnect the nameless in themselves to the nameless in the natural world. The results are phenomenal. They work because they create space for thoughtful, nature-connected moments. In these safe, non-language instants as many as 53 natural attraction senses vibrantly awaken, play, and intensify. No story is present that disrespects them. Additional resonating, trusting, and celebrating activities immediately validate and strengthen each sentient Us-Us connection. This attractive process fills us with nature's nameless beauty, wisdom, and peace. We feel renewed, more colorful, and thankful. As supportive natural attraction feelings reduce our stress, our destructive wants and their accompanying dysfunction and greed wane. They are replaced by attractive nature-connected ideas, stories, and understandings. We revere natural sharing, community, and a greater sensitivity to nature within ourselves, others, and natural areas. We become more environmentally and socially responsible. We feel better.

Ingenuity

Albert Einstein sensed the schism between our stories and the nameless. He said that we experience an optical illusion of consciousness that restrictively separates us from the whole, noting: "The foundation for inner security is...to free ourselves from this prison by widening our circle of compassion, to embrace all living creatures and the whole of nature and its beauty." Significantly, Dr. Einstein did not learn to talk until he was three years old. This means he spent extra non-languaged years with the nameless. Ongoing studies already suggest that strong contacts with Us are a factor held in common by most geniuses. Today, sensory nature-connecting activities foster such contact and our integrity. They enable our culture to nurture the genius of the nameless that lies dormant in each of us.

In the natural world, Us is only found intact in immediate moments in natural areas. The more natural the area, the greater is the intensity of Us. Our indoor environment walls off many aspects of Us. It removes us from connections with sunshine, trees, and fresh air that grow and nurture the nameless in us. However, indoors or outdoors, if we come into a moment with some of our senses non-operant due to lack of use, past assaults or other desensitization stories, we cannot fully know Us in that moment. That may lead to problems. Our injured senses not being able to fully function, enjoy, or register Us is similar to a color blind person not being able to enjoy the natural beauty of the entire color spectrum. To compensate, we may enjoy other attractions with greater intensity.

Connecting with Us in a natural area has the distinct advantage of making a greater fullness and intensity of Us available. In addition, in a natural area Us has greater strength to renew and even regenerate natural senses that have been injured by our divisive nature-conquering stories. For this reason, reconnecting with nature makes sense. It frees and increases higher power because it makes our senses more sensitive and sensible. For example:

> Sandy does the nature activities in this book as part of one of my workshops. By the third hour of the workshop she becomes adept in locating, identifying, and validating her natural attractions to various places in the natural area where the workshop is held. She returns from an activity very excited and explains that she is attracted to the sunlight she sees reflected from the needles of a Douglas Fir tree. She is excited because she sees the reflected light with her left eye, yet she is supposedly "blind" in that eye.

One need only be present once and see or experience this occurrence take place to feel its power. It leads to thinking about what our world might be like if 600 million people had RWN experiences with nature and their community, experiences that were similar to those Sandy had at the workshop. That thought is the essence of the RWN. The sense in it is the love of life; an essence of Sandy, the Douglas Fir, and the spirit of sunlight.

Bonus Activity: Validating Natural Senses and NIAL

Go to an attractive natural area. Ask for its permission to become involved with it, gain its consent to help you with this activity. If the area remains attractive, thank it.

For as long as it feels attractive, go through the list of natural senses in chapter five. Take the time to identify and feel, if possible, each of them in this natural area. Recognize each sense as an ancient, uniquely designed spark of life that resides in the area and in you. Try to feel the wisdom of life each natural sense contains. Let your new-brain story experience the list of senses as a history book of NIAL, of how nature works through attraction relationships. What happens as your new brain becomes conscious of these 53 attraction feelings? Do you feel more supported?

Write down the three most important things you learned from this activity.

Write three green-in-green statements that come from doing this activity.

How would you feel about having your ability to create and enjoy this G/G feeling taken away?

What effect does this activity have on your sense of self-worth?

Appendix D

Well Mind, Well Earth

Well Mind, Well Earth: 109 Environmentally Sensitive Activities for Stress Management, Spirit and Self-esteem by Michael J. Cohen, Ed.D.

Soft Cover, 8 ½" x 11", 260 pages. Includes *The Field Guide to Connecting With Nature: Creating Moments that Let Earth Teach*, the recipient of a 1990 NAI award for excellence in interpretation and part of Vice President Albert Gore's book *Earth In Balance*.

This self-guiding training manual is must reading and doing for anyone who desires to improve their skills in using or teaching the G/O to G/G process. It includes an additional 90 nature reconnecting activities, 25 chapters, and a course syllabus. It lets nature in people and places ecopsychologically fill the natural void in our lives and bridge the many gaps that cause our troubles.

Used independently, or as the text for graduate and undergraduate courses in education and counseling, *Well Mind, Well Earth* enables any student or adult to open new doors to a wide range of environmental and recovery opportunities. Treasured by counselors, educators, and outdoor leaders, this book is the core of Project NatureConnect's Ph.D., M.S., and B.A. independent study degree programs.

In a review in Legacy, the Journal of the National Association for Interpretation, Dr. Daniel Levine, a School Superintendent and first hand observer of the activities says:

"From his decades outdoors, Mike Cohen has devised and collected enjoyable, concise, well-researched nature-connecting activities. In backyards, parks, back country, or even using terrariums, they catalyze lasting, supportive, environmental and interpersonal satisfactions. Each hands-on sensory experience reduces stress and abandonment fears while promoting healthy bonds, minds, and environments. Incorporating these activities in counseling and education allows the natural world and its integrity to become a co-counselor and teacher.

No society has ever established socially and environmentally sound relationships without having strong bonds to the natural world. It is always Mother Earth's dedication, love, and passion for all of life that motivates, guides, and bonds natural beings, including people, to support each other. Without question, *Well Mind, Well Earth* is a book of major significance who's vital contribution deserves our attention. It supplies counselors and educators with tools that let nature nurture."

$58.00 pp. Fifth Edition, World Peace University Press, 1995. Order from:

Project NatureConnect, PO Box 1605, Friday Harbor, WA 98250
Telephone: (360)-378-6313 E-mail: nature@pacificrim.net

Complete information about *Well Mind, Well Earth* and Project NatureConnect can also be found at the Internet World Wide Web site http://www.pacificrim.net/~nature/

Appendix E

References and Bibliography

Cohen, M. J. (1995). Why Don't We Create Moments That Let Earth Teach Us? Cooperative Learning: Vol. 15 No 2 Santa Cruz, CA: International Association for the Study of Cooperation in Education.

Cohen, M. J. (1995). Counseling and Nature: The greening of psychotherapy. Interpsych Newsletter, http://www.pacificrim.net/~nature/counseling.html Also Journal of Humanities and Peace 1996 and ERIC-CASS, U.S. Department of Education.

Cohen, M.J. (1995A). Are You Missing the Missing Link? Proceedings, October, 1994 Conference of the Coalition for Education in the Out Of Doors, P. O. Box 4112, Roche Harbor, Washington: World Peace University Press.

Cohen, M. J. (1994). Well Mind, Well Earth: 107 Environmentally Sensitive Activities for Stress Management, Spirit and Self-Esteem. P. O. Box 4112, Roche Harbor, Washington: World Peace University Press.

Cohen, M. J. (1994a). The Distinguished World Citizen Award: Responsible fulfillment and guidance from nature connections, Taproots. Fall 1994, Cortland NY, Coalition for Education in the Out of Doors.

Cohen, M. J. (1994b). Validations: The experience of connecting with nature, (Tech. Rep. No 21). Roche Harbor WA: World Peace University Press, Department of Integrated Ecology.

Cohen, M. J. (1993). Integrated Ecology: The Process of Counseling With Nature. The Humanistic Psychologist, Vol. 21 No. 3 Washington, DC: American Psychological Association.

Cohen, M. J. (1993B) Counseling with Nature: Catalyzing Sensory Moments that Let Earth Nurture. Counseling Psychology Quarterly, Vol. 6, No. 1, Abingdon Oxfordshire UK: Carfax Publishing.

Cohen, M. J. (1990). Connecting With Nature: Creating Moments That Let Earth Teach. Portland, Oregon: World Peace University Press.

Dossey, L.(1989) Recovering the Soul. New York, New York: Bantam Books.

Farb, P. (1968). Mans Rise to Civilization. New York, New York: Dutton. and MILLENNIUM. (1992) "Mistaken Identity " and "An Ecology of Mind" Public Broadcasting Company TV, National Public Television.

Glendinning, C (1994) My Name is Chellis and I'm in Recovery From Western Civilization: Boston, Shambhala.

Goldman, D. (1993) Psychology's New Interest In the World Beyond the Self, The New York Times New York, NY.

Knapp, C. (1988). Creating Humane Climates Outdoors. Charleston, West Virginia: ERIC/CRESS.

Krutch, J. W. (1954). Voice of the Desert, New York: William Sloane Assoc.

Le Poncin, M. (1990). Brain Fitness. New York: Fawcett Columbine.

Lovelock, J. (1988). The Ages of Gaia. England: Oxford University Press.

Lipkin R. (1995). Bacterial Chatter. Science News, Vol. 147, No. 9 Washington DC: Science Service Inc.

Lipkin, R. (1995) Do Proteins in Cells make Computations? Science News, Vol. 148 July 29 95 Washington DC: Science Service Inc.

Margulis, L. (1986). Microcosmos Four Billion Years of Microbial Evolution. New York, NY: Summit Books.

Monastersky, R. Stute and Thompson (1995). Ice Age Sent Shivers Through the Tropics. Science News, Vol. 148 July 29, 1995 Washington DC: Science Service Inc.

Murchie, G. (1978). Seven Mysteries of Life, Boston, Massachusetts: Houghton Mifflin.

Pearce, J. (1980). Magical Child, New York, New York: Bantam.

Rivlin R., & Gravelle, K. (1984). Deciphering the Senses, New York, New York: Simon and Schuster.

Roszak, T., Gomes M., Kanner A. (1995). Ecopsychology, San Francisco, CA: Sierra Club Books.

Rovee-Collier C. (1992). Infant Memory Shows The Power of Place. Developmental Psychology, March. Quoted in Science News, vol. 141 No. 16 p.244, Washington DC: Science Service Inc.

Sheppard, Paul (1984). Nature and Madness, San Francisco, CA: Sierra Publications.

Spelke, E. (1992). Infants Signal the Birth of Knowledge. Psychological Review, October, 1992 as quoted in Science News, November 14, 1992, Vol. 142 p. 325, Washington DC: Science Service.

Stevens, W. (1993). Want a Room With a View? The New York Times, November 30, New York, NY.

Tsimring, L ((1995) Stressed Bacteria Spawn Elegant Colonies. Science News, Sepember 9,19925, Vol. 148 p. 167, Washington DC: Science Service.

Viscott, D. (1976) The Language of Feelings. New York, NY: Arbor House.

Watson, L. (1988) The Water Planet, New York, New York: Crown Publishers.

Wynne-Edwards (1991). Ecology Denies Darwinism. The Ecologist, May-June, Cornwall, England.